Introductory Speech and Hearing Anatomy and Physiology Workbook

William R. Culbertson
Northern Arizona University

Dennis C. Tanner
Northern Arizona University

Allyn and Bacon
Boston · London · Toronto · Sydney · Tokyo · Singapore

Copyright © 1997 by Allyn & Bacon
A Viacom Company
160 Gould Street
Needham Heights, Massachusetts 02194

Internet: www.abacon.com
America Online: keyword: College Online

ISBN 0-205-26317-8

Printed in the United States of America

10 9 8 7 6 5 4 3 2 1   01 00 99 98 97 96

TABLE of CONTENTS

Introduction v

Unit 1: Introduction to Anatomy   1
         Synopsis of Anatomy and Physiology   3
         Objectives and Study Guide   5
         Study Outline   7
         Self Test   11

Unit 2: Cytology and Histology   13
         Synopsis of Cytology and Histology   15
         Objectives and Study Guide   17
         Study Outline   18
         Self Test   33

Unit 3: The Respiratory System   39
         Synopsis of the Respiratory System   41
         Objectives and Study Guide   43
         Study Outline   45
         Self Test   57

Unit 4: The Phonatory Mechanism   63
         Synopsis of the Phonatory System   65
         Objectives and Study Guide   67
         Study Outline   68
         Self Test   80

Unit 5: The Articulatory Mechanism 89
         Synopsis of the Articulatory System   91
         Objectives and Study Guide   93
         Study Outline   94
         Self Test   119

Unit 6: The Nervous System   129
         Synopsis of the Nervous System   131
         Objectives and Study Guide   135
         Study Outline   136
         Self Test   151

Unit 7: The Auditory System   155
            Synopsis of the Auditory System   157
            Objectives and Study Guide   159
            Study Outline   161
            Self Test   176

Answers to Self Tests   183

References and Recommended Readings   208

INTRODUCTION

The *Introductory Speech and Hearing Anatomy and Physiology Workbook* is intended to augment a one semester (or two quarters) undergraduate course in anatomy and physiology of human communication. Students should regard this material as only one of several training modalities in this field.

The words "anatomy" and "physiology" often intimidate the entry level student. Course titles such as these create thoughts of memorizing long lists of Latin words and trying to comprehend vague concepts of bodily sites and functions. These fears are well-founded if the student tries to absorb advanced material from the start. All too often, the result is an elaborate vocabulary built upon a poor foundation, and the student may feel overwhelmed.

The authors intentionally omitted a large amount of information from the content of these units. This was not because the material was unimportant, but because there is only so much material an undergraduate student should be expected to learn and retain at the introductory level. That is, the purpose of this workbook is to help the student develop a starting point from which to search for additional information as the need arises.

There are many fine texts available in anatomy and physiology that contain important material beyond that which is covered in this workbook. Much or most of it is better advanced to "reference" status. Some additional texts are listed in the reference section.

On top of the need to simplify the material for the student, there is the matter of time. Most communication sciences programs allow one term for anatomy and physiology courses. Professors may find themselves lecturing rapidly, like radio announcers, to include all the material within the time limits of the term. Limitations on the extent of this workbook resulted from many years of full-time clinical and teaching experience.

The units are designed according to a three-step study sequence. First, the student should become familiar with the stated **goals**, and check these again at the completion of the unit. Accomplishment of the goals should provide a very well-rounded idea of anatomy and physiology as it generally applies to the practice of speech-language pathology and audiology.

Next, the student should follow the **study outline**. Study outlines map the course of study, and are arranged to help students reach unit goals. They list important concepts, structures and/or functions, arranged in progressively smaller "chunks," to ease the assimilation of each topic.

These outlines include italicized questions and activities to help the student absorb the material. Space is provided to write the necessary and relevant descriptions, definitions and/or explanations, but the assiduous student may need additional space in a separate notebook. The information required to complete the outlines may come from many sources, including text(s), specimens, models, slides, videos, and lectures. Instructors, of course, may add or delete topics according to course requirements.

Finally, after the student feels comfortable with the material, she or he should take the **self tests**, review the answers, and regard the incorrect ones as feedback on the extent to which the unit is completed. The uses of the self tests are limited by the student's imagination and personal tastes. A student may use the test as a private means of checking study progress, or use them in groups and share the results. The instructor may employ these tests to allow practice in the class, or for reducing anxiety associated with an actual examination. They are valuable learning experience.

The illustrations in this workbook accompany the self tests. Students should fill in the blanks with the names of the structures indicated. Copies of these illustrations are in the section with the answers to the self tests. The authors wish to acknowledge the patience and hard work of Susan Durning and Erica Fuchs in the preparation of these illustrations

A solid background in anatomy and physiology can help the aspiring speech language pathologist or audiologist prepare for the profession in a stimulating and productive way. The purpose of this workbook is to help establish that background. If the study of anatomy and physiology can become more enjoyable through this workbook, then the authors' hopes will have been realized, as well.

UNIT 1
INTRODUCTION TO ANATOMY AND PHYSIOLOGY

Synopsis of Anatomy and Physiology

As students begin the study of anatomy and physiology for speech and hearing, they should absorb some general ideas and basic concepts. The ancient study of the forms and functions of the human body is as rooted in culture as it is in science. Terms and concepts about human life vary with language and philosophy.

The approach of the this workbook is based upon the *Basel Nomina Anatomica*, conceived in 1895, in Basel, Switzerland. This approach represents western European tradition, with terms originally given in Latin. English terms will also appear where they enhance clarity.

Introduction to anatomy and physiology should start with presentations of the disciplines, including their focuses, similarities and differences. Next, the student should examine specializations within each field to gain appreciation for the breadth of study that is possible.

The introductory section presents guidelines for learning the language of anatomy and physiology in the speech and hearing sciences. Terms apply to structures and locations, positions and relationships, processes and actions. Mastery of the information contained in the first unit will provide a solid foundation for mastery of material in future units.

UNIT 1: INTRODUCTION TO ANATOMY
Objectives and Study Guide

The following are the objectives for the unit on the introduction to anatomy and physiology. Success in accomplishing these objectives should prepare the student for further study of the following units. The student can determine mastery of the material presented in unit one by checking the appropriate box as each goal as completed.

1. Differentiate between the sciences of anatomy and physiology.

2. Describe the following subdivisions of anatomy:

    a. descriptive or systemic anatomy
    b. applied or practical anatomy
    c. microscopic anatomy
    d. developmental anatomy
    e. geriatric anatomy

3. Describe the following subdivisions of physiology:

    a. general physiology
    b. applied physiology
    c. experimental physiology
    d. special physiology
    e. pathologic physiology

4. Describe the anatomical position with reference to:

    a. the posture of the body
    b. the position of the limbs
    c. the direction of the eyes
    d. the position of the palms

5. Given diagrams of the human form from different perspectives, identify the following planes:

   a. median or midsagittal plane
   b. sagittal plane
   c. coronal plane
   d. transverse or horizontal plane

6. After defining the following anatomical terms, use them to describe the location of any structure or to compare the locations of two or more structures:

   a. peripheral/central   f. medial/lateral
   b. ventral/dorsal   g. proximal/distal
   c. anterior/posterior   h. caudal/rostral (cranial)
   d. superficial/deep   i. external/internal
   e. superior/inferior

UNIT 1: INTRODUCTION TO ANATOMY and PHYSIOLOGY
Study Outline

I. Definitions
    Fill in the spaces below with the definitions of each science. How do the sciences of anatomy and physiology compliment one another?

    A. Anatomy

    B. Physiology

II. Subdivisions of Anatomy
    Describe each of the following specialized branches in the science of anatomy. Which branches have the most direct relevance to speech-language pathology and audiology?
    A. Descriptive Anatomy

    B. Applied Anatomy

    C. Microscopic Anatomy

    D. Developmental Anatomy

    E. Geriatric Anatomy

III. Subdivisions of Physiology
    Fill in the spaces with your definitions of the following specialized branches of physiology. Describe how each has relevance to the fields of audiology and speech-language pathology.

    A. General Physiology

    B. Applied Physiology

    C. Experimental Physiology

    D. Special Physiology

    E. Pathologic Physiology

IV.   Anatomical Position

A.   Position
In the space provided below, draw a figure of a person facing you and standing in the anatomical position. Why is it important to have a conventional anatomical position?

    1.   Body Standing Erect

    2.   Face Forward

    3.   Arms Extended Downward at Sides

    4.   Palms Forward

B.   Names of Major Topographical Regions
Locate these regions in your drawing.

    1.   Cranial Region

    2.   Cervical Region

    3.   Thoracic Region

    4.   Abdominal Region

    5.   Upper Extremities

    6.   Lower Extremities

V. Anatomical Planes of Reference
    Into which sections do these planes divide the body?

    A. Sagittal

    B. Coronal

    C. Transverse (Horizontal)

VI. Anatomical Location Terms Presented as Antonym (Opposites) Pairs
    In which directions do these terms direct the student?

    A. Peripheral/Central

    B. Ventral/Dorsal

    C. Anterior/Posterior

    D. Superficial/Deep

    E. Superior/Inferior

    F. Medial/Lateral

    G. Proximal/Distal

    H. Caudal/Rostral (Cranial)

    I. External/Internal

UNIT 1: INTRODUCTION TO ANATOMY and PHYSIOLOGY
Self Test

1. The human form, in the anatomical position, is situated with the body posture_____, the palms_____, the eyes_____, the upper extremities_____.

2. The science that studies the functions of living organisms or their parts is _____.

3. The body is divided into anterior and posterior sections by a _____ plane.

4. The body is divided into superior/inferior sections by a _____ plane.

5. The head is _____ to the shoulder.

6. The heel is _____ to the knee.

7. The brain lies inside the skull. The nose is _____ to the brain.

8. The ear lies on the _____ aspect of the skull.

9. The hand is _____ to the elbow.

10. The science that is concerned with the structure of organisms is called _____.

11. The branch of anatomy that deals with the form of the long-lived individual is called _____.

12. The branch of anatomy that deals with the growth of the organism from a single cell to birth is_____ anatomy.

13. The branch of physiology that deals with the changes brought about by the process of disease is _____ physiology.

14. Research in speech/language pathology is primarily studied in _____ physiology.

UNIT 2
CYTOLOGY and HISTOLOGY

Synopsis of Cytology and Histology

Familiarity with the basic components of a system provides a foundation for understanding the larger structure and the scope of its functions. For the biological mechanisms of human communication, the study of cells and tissues is a good place to start.

Elements comprise molecules that, in myriad aggregations, comprise the various proteins. These proteins form the components of cells, and serve the cells' essential functions through their chemical reactions. At some point, the basic elemental substrates become **alive**. The attributes that define life invite the deepest contemplation. Living cells aggregate to form the various **tissues** of which our **organs** are formed. Organs interact and coordinate through **systems** to maintain the complex organism.

The single cell represents the unit constituent of the living body. The human body's genetic code causes proliferation and differentiation of the **zygote**, begun as a single cell product of **gamete** union.

Three basic germ layers appear and become the source for the **four basic tissue types: connective, epithelial, muscle,** and **nervous**. Each type has special properties.

As the **zygote** develops into an **embryo**, discrete structures become visible. Early in fetal development, small arch-shaped ripples appear in its rostral end. These arches are called **branchial arches**. They form the foundations of most of the structures we associate with the peripheral speech and hearing mechanisms.

The human communication mechanism is efficient at its task partly because it is composed of specialized tissues. Special types of connective and epithelial tissues respond to the vibrations of sound energy and air compression to transmit and receive the signals we call speech. Muscle tissue, by virtue of its contractibility, and nervous tissue, through its enhanced excitability, allow the individual to make sounds with the gasses of respiration.

Most books on anatomy and physiology consider the body as divided into convenient sections. This division eases study, but the advanced student will soon learn to appreciate the synergy with which all systems must operate. All **cells, tissues, organs** and **systems** interact to form a unity in the healthy individual.

UNIT 2: CYTOLOGY AND HISTOLOGY
Objectives and Study Guide

The following are the goals for the unit on basic human cells and tissues. The student can determine mastery of the material presented in this unit by checking the appropriate box as each goal as completed.

✓□ 1. Define and give examples of each of these structural units:

        a. cell
        b. tissue
        c. organ
        d. system

✓□ 2. List the qualities that describe the property of life.

✓□ 3. Describe the cell in terms of its basic substance and two principle constituents.

✓□ 4. Name and describe the four basic tissue types of the human body.

✓□ 5. Describe the three germ layers of the developing embryo and major tissues that derive from each.

✓□ 6. Describe branchial arches and the general functions of their derivative structures.

UNIT 2: CYTOLOGY AND HISTOLOGY
Study Outline

I. General Notes
    Fill in the definitions in the spaces below.
    A. Definition of Cytology

    B. Definition of Histology

II. Cytology
    Fill in the cytological definitions in the spaces provided.
    A. Definition of the Cell

    B. Characteristics of Living Matter
        In your own words, describe these characteristics that distinguish living matter from that which is not living.
        1. Characteristics of Life in All Organisms

            a. Growth

            b. Reproduction

            c. Metabolism

            d. Adaptation or Irritability

2. Characteristics of Life in Some Organisms
Define these characteristics. Name some living organisms that do not have these characteristics.

   a. Spontaneous Movement

   b. Expression of Consciousness

   c. Voluntary Use of Senses

C. General Structure of the Cell
Briefly describe the parts and functions of these fundamental cell components.
1. Protoplasm

2. Cytoplasm

3. Nucleus

4. Cell Fluids

5. Cell Shape
What are some common cell shapes? In the boxes below, draw cells of three different shapes.

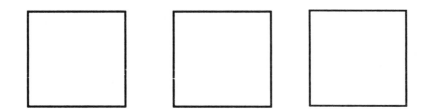

III. Histology
Fill in the fundamental histological definitions in the spaces provided.
   A.   Definition of Tissue

   B.   Four Basic Tissue Types
        Describe the form and function of the following tissue types. What are some examples of each type in the human speech and hearing mechanism?
        1.   Connective

        2.   Epithelial

        3.   Muscle

        4.   Nervous

C.	Connective Tissue
	Describe the following facts about connective tissues in the spaces provided.
	1.	Characteristics of Connective Tissue

		a.	Variability of Intercellular Structure

		b.	Variability of Form

	2.	Functions

		a.	Structural Binding

		b.	Structural Separation

		c.	Fatty Connective Tissue Functions

		d.	Fluid Connective Tissue Functions

3. Types of Connective Tissue
Describe each type of connective tissue. Give examples of each in the human communication mechanism.
   a.   Loose Connective Tissue

      (1)   Areolar Tissue

      (2)   Adipose Tissue

   b.   Dense Connective Tissue

      (1)   Tendons

      (2)   Ligaments

      (3)   Aponeuroses

      (4)   Fascia

   c.   Skeletal Connective Tissue

      (1)   Cartilage

         (a)   Types of Cartilage

            i)   Hyaline

            ii)   Elastic

            iii)   Fibrous

(2) Bone
Describe bone in terms of the special nature of its intercellular material. Describe the following types of bones and give examples of structures containing each.

(a) Long Bone

(b) Short Bone

(c) Flat Bone

(d) Irregular Bone

(3) Articulations of the Skeletal System
What does the term articulation mean in anatomy and physiology? Below are two classication systems for joints. Describe the extent of movement each joint allows. What are the advantages of each type? Give examples of each type of joint in the human communication mechanism.

(a) Functional Classification of Joints

i) Synarthrodial

ii) Amphiarthrodial

iii) Diarthrodial

(4) Anatomical Classification of Joints
Describe the following anatomical joint types. To what functional classification does each correspond?

(a) Fibrous

(b) Cartilaginous

(c) Synovial

d. Divisions of the Skeletal System
What structures comprise these skeletal divisions.
(1) Axial Skeleton

(2) Appendicular Skeleton

4. Fluid Connective Tissue
    What characteristic of the intercellular structure of fluid connective tissue distinguishes it? What are the functions of the two fluid tissues?

    a. Blood

    b. Lymph

D. Epithelial Tissue

    1. Characteristics of Epithelial Tissue
        Describe these aspects of epithelial tissue in the spaces provided.
        a. Intercellular Structure

        b. Cellular Arrangement

    2. Functions of Epithelial Tissue

        a. Protective

        b. Absorptive

        c. Secretory

        d. Glandular

        e. Sensory

3. Types of Epithelial Tissue
Describe these types of epithelial tissue. Where might they be found within the mechanism for communication?
   a.   Proper Epithelium

   b.   Mesothelium

   c.   Endothelium

   d.   Descriptive Terms
        Define some terms that classify epithelial tissue.
        (1)   Cell Shape

              (a)   Squamous

              (b)   Columnar

              (c)   Pyramidal

              (d)   Cuboidal

        (2)   Layers

              (a)   Simple

              (b)   Stratified

E.   Muscle Tissue
     Describe muscle tissue in terms of the following.
     1.   Characteristics

     2.   Function
          Describe how muscle tissue functions at these progressively
          larger contractile units.

          a.   Sarcomere

          b.   Myofibril

          c.   Muscle Fiber

          d.   Muscle Fasciculus

          e.   Muscle

     3.   Types of Muscle Tissue
          Describe each type. Where is each type of muscle tissue
          found?
          a.   Smooth

          b.   Cardiac

          c.   Striated

     4.   Muscle Feedback
          What is the role of conscious and unconscious muscle
          feedback in the regulation of muscle function for speech?

5. Muscle Attachment
   To which end of a muscle do the following tems refer?
   a.   Origin

   b.   Insertion

6. Muscle Function Terminology
   Define the following muscle function terms.

   a.   Flexion

   b.   Extension

   c.   Adduction

   d.   Abduction

7. Names of Muscles
   Give examples of muscles named according to the characteristics below.

   a.   Shape

   b.   Function

   c.   Location

F.   Nervous Tissue
Describe the following special features of nervous tissue.
1.   Characteristics

a.   Excitability

b.   Conductivity

2.   Functions

a.   Excitatory

b.   Inhibitory

3.   Types of Nervous Tissue
a.   Neurons
Describe the following types of neurons. Give examples of locations at which each may be found in the mechanism for human communication. In the boxes provided, draw stylized representations of each type and label the cell body, axons and dendrites.
(1)   Unipolar Neurons

(2)   Bipolar Neurons

(3)   Multipolar Neurons

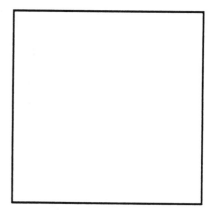

b.   Neuroglial Cells
Describe the following neuroglial cells. What are their unique functions?

(1)   Oligodendrocytes

(2)   Astrocytes

(3)   Microglia

(4)   Neurilemma

G. Tissue Differentiation
Define each of the following germ layers in the spaces provided.
Give Examples of organs or structures in the speech or hearing
mechanism derived from each.
1. Germ Layers

a. Endoderm (Entoderm)

b. Mesoderm

c. Ectoderm

2. Branchial Arches
What is a branchial arch? At which end of the embryo do they
appear? List the speech and hearing structures that develop
from each arch in the spaces provided.

a. Mandibular Arch

b. Hyoid Arch

c. Third Branchial Arch

d. Fourth Branchial Arch

e. Fifth Branchial Arch

f. Sixth Branchial Arch

IV.   Organs and Systems

    A.   Definitions
        Define the following in the spaces provided.

        1.   System

        2.   Organ

    B.   Review of Systems and Their Interactions
        What are the life sustaining functions of the following systems?
        Which ones have overlaid communicative functions?

        1.   Respiratory

        2.   Nervous

        3.   Muscular

        4.   Circulatory

        5.   Digestive

        6.   Urinary

        7.   Endocrine

        8.   Vascular

        9.   Skeletal

        10.   Integumentary

        11.   Articular

UNIT 2: CYTOLOGY AND HISTOLOGY
Self Test

1. A cell is composed of_____.

2. Four characteristics that identify an entity as being alive are:
    a. _____
    b. _____
    c. _____
    d. _____

3. The study of collections of cells that have similar structures and functions is called _____.

4. The thicker part of the protoplasm of a cell is called the _____.

5. Name the tissue types that have the following special characteristics:
    a. Characterized by irritability_____.
    b. Forms a protective sheath covering the interior and exterior surfaces of the body _____.
    c. Mediates body movements by virtue of contractile properties _____.
    d. Binds the body structures together and aids in body maintenance _____.
    e. Conducts changes in electrical potential _____.

6. Indicate from which germ layers the following structures are derived:
    a. The brain _____.
    b. The muscles of the tongue _____.
    c. The cranial nerves _____.
    d. The jaw bone _____.
    e. The lungs _____.

7. The branchial skeleton includes the _____ and _____ bones, as well as the _____and _____ cartilages.

8. The primary function of the branchial and hypobranchial musculature is _____.

9. Embryonic cells differentiate into three distinct groups called_____ _____ .

10. Joints that move freely are called _____ or _____.

11. The type of muscle that is under voluntary control is _____.

12. What comprises a *motor unit*? _____.

13. The term applied to the attachment of a muscle to a more moveable body part is _____.

14. Define *organ*. _____
    _____ .

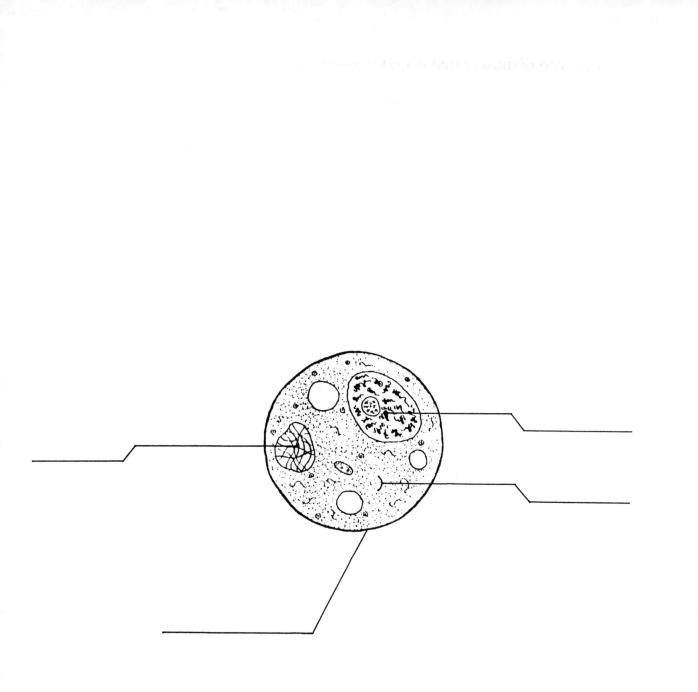

SOMATIC CELL

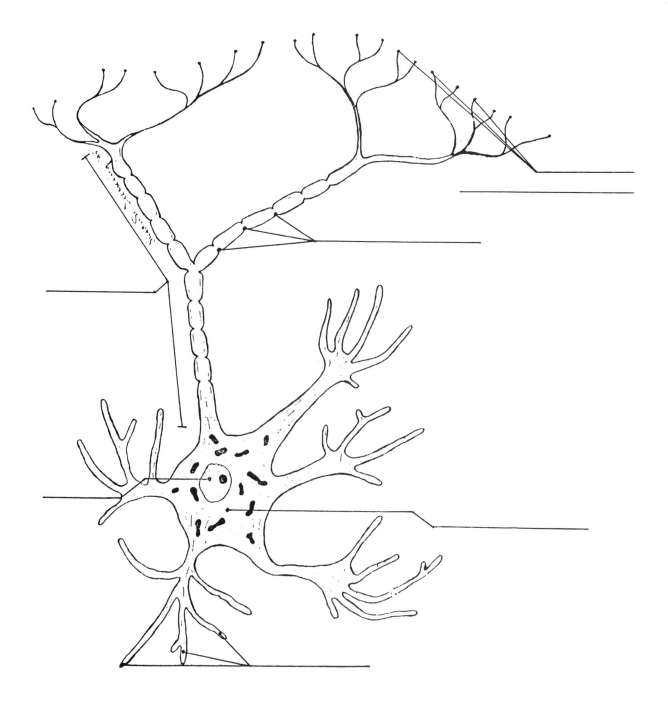

NEURON

UNIT 3
THE RESPIRATORY MECHANISM

Synopsis of the Respiratory System

The essential function of the respiratory system is to allow the exchange of gasses to and from the environment. By virtue of its specialized structure, the respiratory mechanism allows the exchange of **oxygen** from the external atmosphere for **carbon dioxide** from the bloodstream. While the life function of respiration is automatic, human beings have learned to control the respiratory system for the overlaid function of speaking.

The phase in which air flows into the lungs is referred to as **inspiration**. Air, and other liquids and gases, flow from higher pressure regions to lower pressure regions. An inward flow of oxygen containing atmospheric air results from contraction of the muscles of inhalation. More than a dozen muscles are involved in this process. Contractions of these muscles increase the size of the thorax vertically, anteroposteriorly and transversely. As the size of the thorax increases, the pressure inside decreases according to **Boyle's Law**. Certain forces that oppose inspiration must be overcome. They include the small resistance to air flow in the respiratory airway the resistance to deformation of the respiratory tissue or the elastic recoil of the lungs and thorax, and the fluid pressure of the abdomen.

Expiration is the phase in which air flows from the lungs. This flow is caused by a decrease in the dimensions of the thorax and a resulting increase in its internal pressure. Expiratory changes are normally effected by allowing the forces that oppose inspiration to act. At the peak of inspiration, the alveolar pressure is equal to the atmospheric pressure. When the muscles of inspiration relax, the alveolar pressure exceeds that of the atmosphere and causes air to flow out of the lungs. When forceful expulsion of respiratory air is required, the muscles of expiration contract.

The anatomy of the healthy respiratory mechanism creates a dynamic balance among the structures of the torso. The torso, or the body without the extremities, is divided into superior and inferior divisions by the dome shaped **diaphragm**. The diaphragm is also the primary muscle of inhalation. The superior division of the torso, containing the heart, lungs, ribs and muscles, is called the **thorax**. The inferior division is the **abdomen**. This fluid-filled cavity contains the digestive system and various organs and glands. Function of the muscles of respiration alternately shifts the balance of internal and external pressures between and among the thoracic cavities and the external atmosphere.

Viewing the respiratory system as a **biological pump** is a convenient analogy. This pump compresses the air used for vital functions and for speech purposes. Physiological terms for respiratory pressures include **alveolar pressure** or pressure within the lungs and **pleural pressure** or pressure within the thorax but outside the lungs. **Abdominal pressure** is the pressure in the abdomen.

The volumes or air involved in respiratory functions are measured with a spirometer. **Tidal capacity** is the total volume of air expired during each normal respiratory cycle. **Complemental air** is the maximum volume of air that can be inspired beyond normal inhalation and is also known as inspiratory reserve. **Supplemental air**, or expiratory reserve volume, is the maximum volume of air that can be expired beyond the end of a normal tidal expiration. **Residual air** volume is the air remaining in the lungs that cannot be exhaled. **Vital capacity** is the total volume of air measurable within the lungs and includes the sum of tidal capacity, complemental air and supplemental air. Respiratory rates vary with age and activity. Sleep may decrease the rate by as much as twenty-five percent.

Respiration for speech is normally a voluntary act, while vegetative breathing is an autonomic function. For speaking, the muscles of the thorax decrease the air pressure inside the lungs at a rate much quicker than that for quiet breathing. This results in a quick inhalation. Then the muscles slowly relax, so the gas inside the lungs will last longer. The speech segment will be longer.

The pressurized gas from the lungs flows upward to power the larynx and create the other sound sources for speech. Without the power provided by the respiratory system, speech would be a series of oral gestures, accompanied by very little sound.

The respiratory pump provides a driving force for the generation of voiced and unvoiced sounds. It provides the energy necessary for a series of valving events that result in the acoustic characteristics of phonemes. Voluntary respiratory behavior plays an important role in the suprasegmental aspects of speech, including loudness, pitch, emphasis and pauses.

UNIT 3: THE RESPIRATORY SYSTEM
Objectives and Study Guide

Successful accomplishment of these objectives should give the student a basic understanding of respiratrory function in speech production. It should also provide the foundation with which to apply the facts to the evaluation and treatment of speech disorders. When the objective is accomplished, the student should check the box beside each objective.

1. Describe two definitions of respiration.

2. Describe the mechanics of physical respiration in terms of the principles of Boyle's law.

3. Describe the structures and divisions of the upper and lower respiratory tracts.

4. Describe the skeleton of the thorax and abdomen.

5. Describe the mechanics and purposes of respiration for life and for speech.

6. Describe the muscles of inhalation and their functions.

7. Differentiate between the muscles of inhalation and the muscles of exhalation.

8. Describe the following respiratory volumes:

   a. Tidal Volume

   b. Vital Capacity

   c. Inspiratory Reserve

   d. Expiratory Reserve.

   e. Residual Volume

✐☐ 9. Describe the different respiratory patterns, including:

       a. Diaphragmatic/Abdominal   d. Cheyne-Stokes

       b. Thoracic   e. Neurogenic Hyperventilation

       c. Clavicular   f. Kussmaul Respiration

✐☐ 10. Describe chronic diseases of the respiratory tract, including asthma, emphysema, and chronic bronchitis.

UNIT 3: THE RESPIRATORY SYSTEM
Study Outline

I. Two Definitions for Respiration.
Fill in the definitions in the spaces provided. Why do we describe respiration in two ways?

    A.   Physical

         1.   Biological Function

         2.   Overlaid Function

    B.   Chemical
Write the chemical equation for respiration.

II. Structures of the Respiratory Tract

    A.   Location of the Respiratory System
Describe the general location of the structures for breathing. Which ones are located in the upper part?

         1.   Upper Respiratory Tract

         2.   Lower Respiratory Tract

B.   Skeleton of the Respiratory Tract

  1.   Spinal Column

    a.   Vertebrae

      (1)   Structure
              Describe the general structure of a vertebra.

      (2)   Types of Vertebrae

        (a)   Cervical

            i)   Special Names for Cervical
                   Vertebrae
                   *To which vertebrae do these names
                   refer?*

                a)   Atlas

                b)   Axis

                c)   Vertebra Prominens

        (b)   Thoracic

        (c)   Lumbar

        (d)   Sacral

        (e)   Coccygeal

  2.   Pelvic Girdle
         What is the role of the pelvic girdle in respiration?

3. Rib Cage

    a. Ribs

    b. Sternum

4. Clavicles

5. Scapulae

C. Nose and Nasal Cavity

1. Nares

2. Septum

3. Root

4. Choanae

D. Pharynx
Differentiate between these subdivisions of the pharynx.

1. Nasopharynx

2. Oropharynx

3. Laryngopharynx

E. Oral Cavity Structure and Function
Describe the locations of these oral landmarks.

1. Fauces

2. Triangular Fossa

3. Tonsils

F. Laryngopharynx
What is the respiratory function of the larynx?

G. Trachea
    Describe the structure and location of the trachea. What is its location relative to the esophagus?

H. Bronchial Tree

    1. Main Stem Bronchi

    2. Secondary Bronchi

    3. Tertiary Bronchi

    4. Bronchioles

I. Lungs
    Describe the following structures and characteristics of the lungs in the spaces provided.

    1. Right and Left Lung Differences

    2. Alveoli

    3. Pleurae

        a. Intrapleural Fluid

        b. Visceral Pleura

        c. Parietal Pleura

III. Mechanics of Respiration
      How does Boyle's law relate to breathing?

A.   Boyle's Law

B.   Inspiration and Expiration

1.   Respiratory Cycle
Define a respiratory cycle. What is the normal I-Fraction (ratio of the duration of inhalation to the duration of the entire cycle) for quiet breathing? Describe the differences between the respiratory cycle for speech and that for quiet breathing.

a.   Vegetative Breathing.

b.   Respiration for Speech

2.   Respiratory Rates
What are normal rates for and adult, child and for an infant? How are these rates measured?

a.   Adult Respiratory Rate Range

b.   Child Respiratory Rate Range

c.   Infant Respiratory Rate Range

3. Respiratory Patterns
Describe the most commonly encountered patterns of respiration? How does the diagnostician identify one? Is there one pattern that is more efficient?

a. Normal Patterns of Respiration

(1) Diaphragmatic/Abdominal

(2) Thoracic

(3) Clavicular

b. Pathological Patterns of Respiration
Describe these pathological patterns of respiration.
(1) Cheyne-Stokes Respiration

(2) Neurogenic Hyperventilation

(3) Kussmaul Respiration

C.   Muscles of Respiration

1.   Function of the Muscles of Respiration
      *How do the following movements bring about changes in
      thoracic volumes?*

      a.   Diaphragmatic Movement

      b.   Costal Movement

            (1)   Pump Handle

            (2)   Bucket Handle

2.   Inhalation: Active Movement

      a.   Primary Muscles of Inhalation
            Describe the origins and insertions of these muscles.

            (1)   Diaphragm

            (2)   External Intercostals

b. Secondary Muscles of Inhalation
Under what conditions will an individual employ these muscles? Describe their origins and insertions.

    (1)   Pectoralis Majorus/Minoris

    (2)   Costal Levators

        (a)   12 paired

        (b)   C-7 to T-11

    (3)   Serratus Anteriorus

    (4)   Serratus Posterior Superiorus

    (5)   Latissimus Dorsi

    (6)   Scalenus

        (a)   C-3 thru. C-6

        (b)   To Ribs 1 & 2

3.   Exhalation
     Describe the different manners in which gas is expelled from the respiratory system.

   a.   Passive Movement

   b.   Active Movement

     (1)   Muscles of Exhalation
           What is the role of the muscles of expiration in the production of speech?

           (a)   Primary Muscles of Expiration
                 Describe the origins and insertions of these muscles.

                 i)   Internal Intercostals

                 ii)   Rectus Abdominus

                 iii)   Transversus Abdominus

                 iv)   External Obliques

                 v)   Internal Obliques

(b)   Secondary Muscles of Expiration
Describe the origins and insertions of the secondary muscles of exhalation. Under what circumstances might they be employed?

i)   Serratus Posterior Inferiorus

ii)   Quadratus Lumborum

iii)   Subcostals

iv)   Latissimus Dorsi

IV. Measurement of Respiratory Function
What are the implications of respiratory function testing in the evaluation and treatment of communicative disorders?

A. Spirometry
Describe the spirometer. Can a speech-language pathologist estimate respiratory efficiency for speech without instrumentation? If so, how?

B. Volumes
Define the following respiratory volumes. What are normal values?

1. Vital Capacity

2. Tidal

3. Inspiratory Reserve (Complimentary)

4. Expiratory Reserve (Supplementary)

5. Residual

V. Diseases of the Respiratory System
    Describe these common chronic diseases of respiration. What limitations might be imposed of the effects of speech therapy for individuals suffering from these conditions?

    A. Chronic Obstructive Pulmonary Disease ("C.O.P.D.")

    B. Asthma

    C. Emphysema

    D. Chronic Bronchitis

UNIT 3: RESPIRATORY SYSTEM
Self Test

1. What are the two points of view from which we can describe respiration? _____ and _____.

2. Air moves in and out of the respiratory tract coincident with changes in the _____ of the thorax in a manner consistent with which law of physics? _____.

3. Identify the following anatomical structures as belonging to either the *upper* or *lower* respiratory tract.

   a. Nasopharynx _____   f. Bronchi _____

   b. Lungs _____   g. Pleurae _____

   c. Oral Cavity _____   h. Nostrils _____

   d. Fauces _____   I. Trachea _____

   e. Choanae _____   j. Oropharynx _____

4. The *non-biological* function of respiration is_____.

5. The respiratory system consists of_____.

6. A respiratory cycle consists of _____.

7. The normal respiratory rate for adults is_____.

8. The operation of Boyle's law is assured by action of_____.

9. The primary muscles of inhalation are _____.

10. During normal exhalation, the muscles of respiration _____.

11. The first seven vertebrae are called _____.

12. The lateral movement of ribs 7-10 is referred to as_____.

13. The muscles of exhalation contract for _____
    _____.

14. The true ribs attach anteriorly to the _____.

15. A device which measures respiratory volumes is called a
    _____.

16. The vertebrae closest to the lungs are called _____.

17. The volume of air inhaled and exhaled during any single expiratory
    cycle is called the_____.

18. The quantity of air that can be exhaled after as deep an inhalation as
    possible is called_____.

19. The I-fraction for speech is approximately _____.

20. Expiratory reserve is also known as _____, and is the
    term used to describe the volume of air that _____
    _____.

21. The two *normal* patterns of respiration are called _____
    _____.

22. Describe Cheyne-Stokes respiration _____
    _____.

23. What are the rehabilitation implications of C.O.P.D? _____
    _____

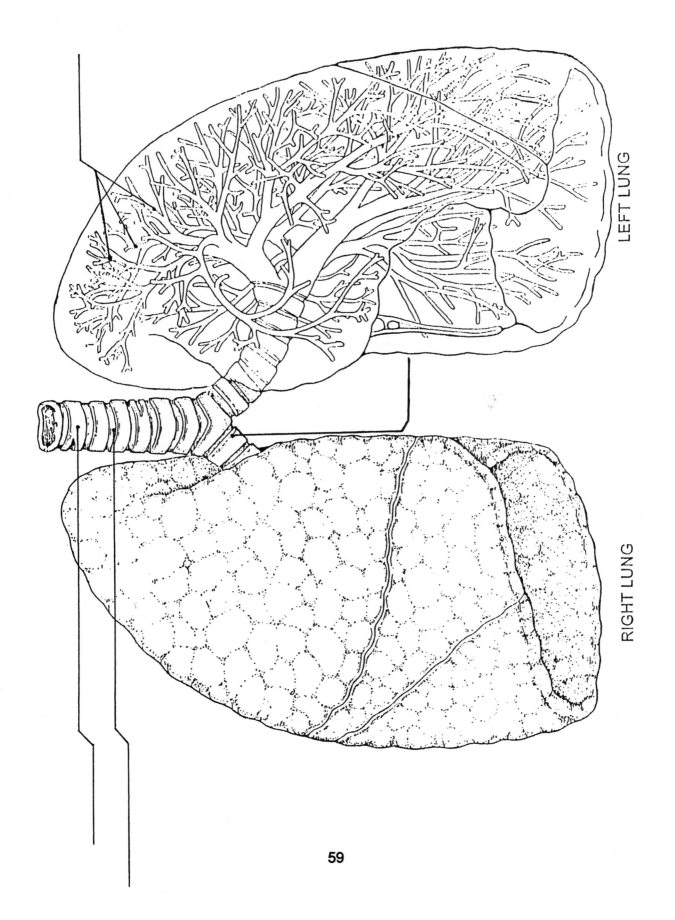

LEFT LUNG

RIGHT LUNG

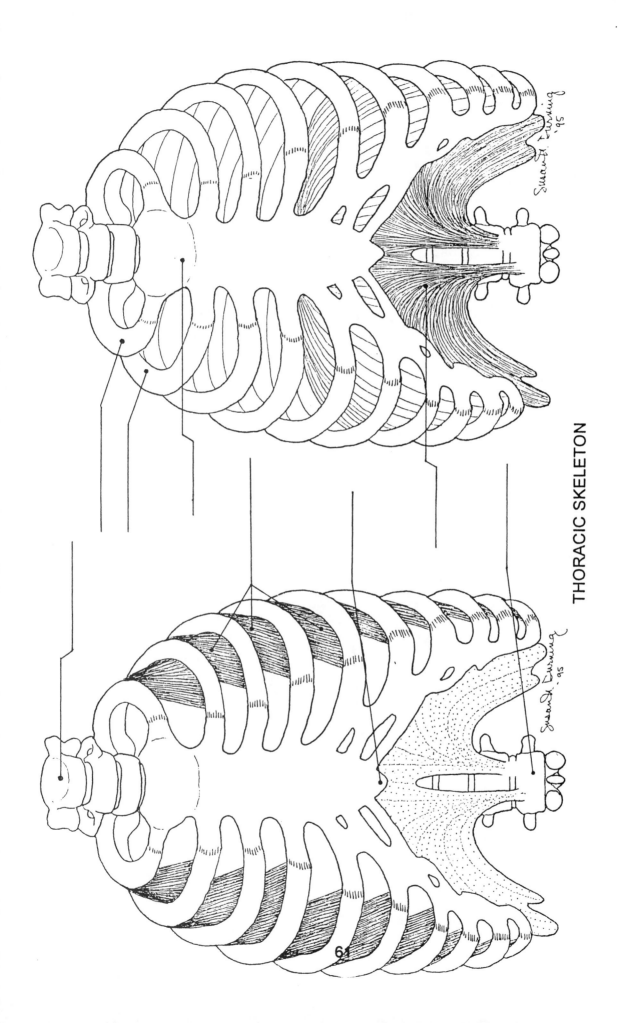

THORACIC SKELETON

61

UNIT 4
THE PHONATORY MECHANISM

Synopsis of the Phonatory Mechanism

The production of speech depends on the transmission of sound waves. One of the main anatomical locations for sound production is the **larynx**. The larynx functions as a valve. Because both food traveling to the stomach and air passing to the lungs begin in the same passage, the larynx serves a dual purpose. It permits the passage of air to and from the lungs while being capable of closing during swallowing to protect the lungs from food and other foreign bodies. The opening at the level of the vocal folds is called the **glottis**. Other functions of the larynx include stabilization of the thorax for body exertions and regulation of airflow in and out of the lungs. **Phonation** refers to any type of vibratory sound produced at the level of the larynx. Whisper is also a function of partially contracting the vocal folds.

The larynx consists of nine **cartilages** of which three are paired. The largest is the **thyroid cartilage**. The **cricoid cartilage** resembles a signet ring. The **epiglottis**, which is not vital to humans, snaps down like a trap to help protect the airways. The **arytenoids**, **corniculates** and **cuneiforms** are the paired cartilages.

The cartilages of the larynx are tied to one another by **intrinsic ligaments**. **Extrinsic ligaments** connect the laryngeal cartilages to the hyoid bone, above, and to the first tracheal ring, below. In addition to their functions as connecting tissues, the intrinsic laryngeal ligaments, spread thin in some places to form membranes, play a role in producing the vibrations we associate with the voice.

The musculature of the phonatory mechanism moves its structure to adjust its openings and postures. **Intrinsic laryngeal muscles** have both origin and insertion within the laryngeal structure. They are primary to pitch and loudness control. Only one muscle is responsible for opening, or abducting, the vocal folds: the posterior cricoarytenoid. Adductors are intrinsic muscles responsible for forcefully closing the vocal folds. Tensors and relaxers work to elongate and shorten the vocal folds. **Extrinsic laryngeal muscles** have one connection outside the larynx and are frequently referred to as either suprahyoid or infrahyoid. Suprahyoid muscles help elevate the larynx while infrahyoids (neck strap muscles) are involved in lowering it.

The larynx comprises a portion of the pharynx. This portion is called the **laryngopharynx**. It is divided into three cavities. At the superior end in the vestibular portion. This is the entrance to the airway. The middle division of the laryngopharynx is the ventricle. It is bordered by two sets of tissue folds: the **ventricular (false) vocal folds** at the superior end and the **(true) vocal folds** at the inferior end. Inferior to the ventricle is the **subglottic area** of the laryngopharynx.

The act of producing voiced speech is dependent on respiratory support. The vocal folds rapidly vibrate as the compressed respiratory air travels over their surfaces. The vocal folds are capable of closing rapidly due both **myoelastic** properties of the laryngeal tissue and the **aerodynamic** Bernoulli principle. Pitch and loudness are a result of fine regulation and coordination between subglottic air pressure and muscle resistance. During elevation of pitch, the mass per unit length of the vocal folds is decreased. Lowering of the pitch is a result of an increase of mass per unit length of the vocal folds. To effect these mass changes, the vocalis muscle and the vocal ligament are adjusted by fine movements of the arytenoid cartilages which are capable of sliding and rotating in response to intrinsic muscle tension and length.

UNIT 4: THE PHONATORY MECHANISM
Objectives and Study Guide

Mastery of the following objectives should give the student a basic understanding of the form and function of the mechanism we use to produce the voice. Such an understanding will give the student a point of departure for study of the evaluation and treatment of phonatory disorders. Students should check the boxes by the objectives as they accomplish them.

✎☐ 1. Describe the larynx in terms of its physical appearance, location, and functions.

✎☐ 2. Describe the general process of phonation and the glottic cycle.

✎☐ 3. Describe glottal postures and their effects on phonatory source characteristics.

✎☐ 4. Name and identify the major cartilages of the larynx.

✎☐ 5. Describe the articulations of the major laryngeal cartilages.

✎☐ 6. Name and identify the major ligaments and membranes of the larynx.

✎☐ 7. Name and identify the intrinsic muscles of the larynx.

✎☐ 8. Name and identify the three sections of the cavity of the larynx.

✎☐ 9. Differentiate the functions of the intrinsic versus the extrinsic muscles of the larynx.

UNIT 4: THE PHONATORY MECHANISM
Study Outline

I. General Structure and Function

    A. General Description and Location
        Describe the larynx and its general location.

    B. Evolution
        What is the function of the larynx in lower animals?

    C. Biological Function
        What are the functions of the laryngeal valve have apart from phonation?

    D. Speech Function
        What is the speech function of the larynx? How does it accomplish this function?

        1. The Glottis and Vocal Folds
            What is the glottis? Differentiate between abduction and adduction of the vocal folds.

            a. Abduction

            b. Adduction

2.	Physiology of Normal Phonation

a.	The Glottic Cycle
Describe the following phases of the glottic cycle: closed phase, opening phase, closing phase.
(1)	Closed Phase

(2)	Opening Phase

(3)	Closing Phase

(4)	Forces
Describe the forces at work during the glottic cycle.
(a)	Myoelastic

(b)	Aerodynamic

b.	Glottal Frequency
What are the effects of changes in glottal frequency?
(1)	Average Glottal Frequency

(a)	Males

(b)	Females

(2)	Mechanism for Changing Glottal Frequency
How do the vocal folds change as pitch increases? How are these changes brought about?

c.	Glottal Cycle Amplitude
Describe the changes that occur in the glottal cycle as the voice becomes louder.

II.   The Framework of the Larynx:

A.   The Hyoid Bone
Is the hyoid bone part of the larynx?

1.   Structure

a.   Corpus

b.   Greater Cornua

c.   Lesser Cornua

2.   Function of the Hyoid Bone
a. Attachments

b. Relationship to Tongue and to Larynx

B. Cartilages of the Larynx
What types of cartilages form the skeleton of the larynx?

    1.   Unpaired Cartilages of the Larynx
        a. Thyroid Cartilage
        Describe the Thyroid Cartilage. What is its size relative to the other laryngeal cartilages?

            (1)   Structure
                (a)   Laminae
                Describe the angle of fusion of the thyroid laminae. How does this angle change as the individual develops? Is there any relationship between this angle and the sound of the voice?

                (b)   Cornua

        b.   Cricoid Cartilage
        What are the superior and inferior attachments of the cricoid cartilage?

            (1)   Attachments

            (2)   Structure
                (a)   Lamina

                (b)   Arch

                (c)   Articular Surface

c.   Epiglottis
Describe the following structures in the spaces below.

(1)   Structure and Location

(2)   Attachments of the Epiglottis

(3)   Glossoepiglottic Folds

(a)   Epiglottic Valleculae

(b)   Laryngeal inlet

(4)   Epiglottitis
Why is epiglottitis a life threatening condition?

2. Paired Cartilages of the Larynx
   a. Arytenoid Cartilages
   Describe the following aspects of the arytenoid cartilages.

   (1) Structure

       (a) Vocal processes

       (b) Muscular processes

   (2) Function
   Describe the cricoarytenoid joint. What type of joint is it?

       (a) Adduction/Abduction
       Describe the following movements of the arytenoid cartilages.
       i) Rotation

       ii) Gliding or Sliding

       iii) Tilting

(b) Cartilaginous Glottis
How much of the glottis is bordered by tissue with underlying cartilage? What are the physiological implications of this fact?

b. Minor Cartilages of the Larynx
Describe the locations of these minor cartilages.

    (1) Corniculate cartilages

    (2) Cuneiform cartilages

    (3) Triticeal cartilages

C.   Ligaments of the Larynx
Describe the attachments of these ligaments. What are their functions? What differentiates an intrinsic *ligament from an* extrinsic *ligament?*

1.   Extrinsic Ligaments

a.   Thyrohyoid Ligament

b.   Cricotracheal Ligament

2.   Intrinsic Ligaments

a.   Cricothyroid
Why is the cricothyroid ligament called the most important intrinsic ligament?

b.   Conus Elasticus

c.   Cricovocal Membrane
Describe the Vocal Ligament. What are its anterior and posterior attachments? How does it relate to the cricovocal membrane?

d.   Vestibular Ligament

III. Articulations of the Larynx

    A.   Cricothyroid Articulation
          Describe the articulation of the thyroid cartilage with the cricoid cartilage.
          1.   Rotation About the Horizontal Axis
               What effect does this motion have on the pitch of the voice?

          2.   Gliding

    B.   Cricoarytenoid Articulation
          Review cricoarytenoid articulation
          1.   Rotation

          2.   Gliding or Sliding (Anterior/Posterior and Lateral/Medial)

          3.   Tilting

IV. Cavities of the Larynx (Laryngopharynx)
Describe these divisions of the laryngopharynx.
    A.   Vestibular (Superior) Division

          1.   Extends from Inlet to Ventricular Folds

          2.   Epiglottis

          3.   Aryepiglottic Folds

               Draw a diagram representing the cross section of the laryngeal cavity in the box on the right.

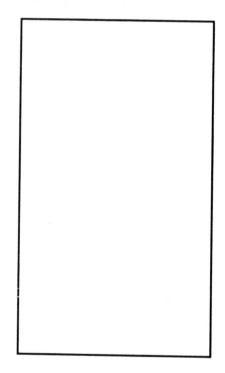

B.   Ventricular (Middle Division)

    a.   From Ventricular (Vestibular) Folds to Vocal Folds

    b.   Ventricular Folds
Is it possible to adduct the ventricular folds?

        (1)   Composition

        (2)   Attachments

    c.   Vocal Folds
Describe these aspects of the vocal folds. Why are these folds called the true *vocal folds?*

        (1)   Composition

           (a)   Thyroarytenoid Muscles

           (b)   Vocalis Muscles

           (c)   Vocal Ligaments

        (2)   Attachments of the Vocal Folds

        (3)   Glottis
Draw a diagram of the glottis as seen from above. Show which part is intercartilaginous.

           (a)   Intermembranous

           (b)   Intercartilaginous

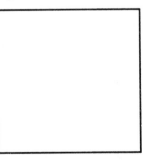

C.   Infraglottic (Subglottic) Division
What is the relationship of subglottic air pressure to voice loudness?

V. **Muscles of the Larynx: Intrinsic and Extrinsic**

A. **Intrinsic Muscles of the Larynx**
Why are these muscles referred to as intrinsic? *What is the general function of the intrinsic muscles of the larynx? Describe the origins/insertions and functions of these muscles in the spaces provided.*

1. **Muscles That Control Tension/Length of the Vocal Ligament**

   a. Cricothyroid

   b. Thyroarytenoid

   c. Vocalis

2. **Muscles That Control Glottal Aperture**

   a. Posterior Cricoarytenoid

   b. Lateral Cricoarytenoid

   c. Transverse Arytenoid

   d. Oblique Arytenoid

3. **Muscles That Modify Laryngeal Inlet**

   a. Aryepiglottic

   b. Thyroepiglottic

   c. Ventricular

B.   Extrinsic Muscles of the Larynx
Why are these muscles described as extrinsic? How would you describe the general function of the extrinsic muscles of the larynx? Describe the origins/insertions and the functions of the extrinsic muscles in the spaces provided.

1.   Suprahyoid Muscles

a.   Digastric

b.   Stylohyoid

c.   Mylohyoid

d.   Geniohyoid

e.   Hyoglossus

2.   Infrahyoid

a.   Sternohyoid

b.   Omohyoid

c.   Thyroid

d.   Sternothyroid

3.   Indirect Displacers of the Larynx

a.   Palatopharyngeus

b.   Stylopharyngeus

c.   Inferior Pharyngeal Constrictor

UNIT 4: THE PHONATORY MECHANISM
Self Test

1. What is the most important biological function of the larynx?
   _____.

2. The trachea is (posterior/anterior) to the esophagus.

3. What is the secondary or overlaid function of the larynx?
   _____.

4. Describe the voice in physiological terms. _____
   _____.

5. The perceived pitch of the voice is related to_____
   _____.

6. The perceived loudness of the voice is related to what physiological
   phenomenon? _____.

7. Describe the glottis. _____.

8. The hyoid bone is classified as a part of the _____.

9. The largest cartilage of the larynx is the _____.

10. The lowest cartilage of the larynx is the _____.

11. The flat parts of the thyroid and cricoid cartilages are called the _____.

12. The laryngeal prominence marks location of the _____.

13. The cartilage that is shaped like a signet ring is the _____.

14. The vocal ligaments are attached posteriorly to what structures? _____
    _____.

15. Movement of the vocal folds away from the midline is called _____.

16. The muscles that tense and lengthen the vocal ligaments are the
    a. posterior arytenoid muscles.
    b. suprahyoid muscles.
    c. transverse arytenoid and oblique arytenoid muscles.
    d. cricothyroid, thyroarytenoid, and vocalis muscles.

17. Which of the following muscles do not adduct the vocal folds.
    a. posterior cricoarytenoid muscles.
    b. lateral cricoarytenoid muscles.
    c. oblique arytenoid muscles.
    d. transverse arytenoid muscle.

18. The lateral and posterior cricoarytenoid muscles attach to the arytenoid cartilages at which structures? _____
    _____.

19. During heavy breathing, the vocal folds what position do the vocal folds assume? _____.

20. Of what kind of joint is the cricoarytenoid joint an example? _____.

21. The upper free border of the cricothyroid membrane is called the _____
    _____.

22. What distinguishes the intrinsic muscles of the larynx from the extrinsic muscles? _____
    _____.

23. Which muscle pair abducts the vocal ligaments? _____.

24. What are the main functions of the extrinsic muscles of the larynx?
    _____.

25. What term is used to describe the air pressure inferior to the adducted vocal folds? _____.

26. What is the average glottal frequency in adult females? _____

27. Describe the forces that, according to currently held theories, act to close the glottis during phonation. _____

_____

_____

_____

_____

_____

_____.

28. Which muscles make up the vocal folds? _____ & _____.

29. In which direction does the thyroid cartilage move during deglutition? _____.

30. What role do the valleculae play in the evaluation of deglutition?

_____

_____

_____.

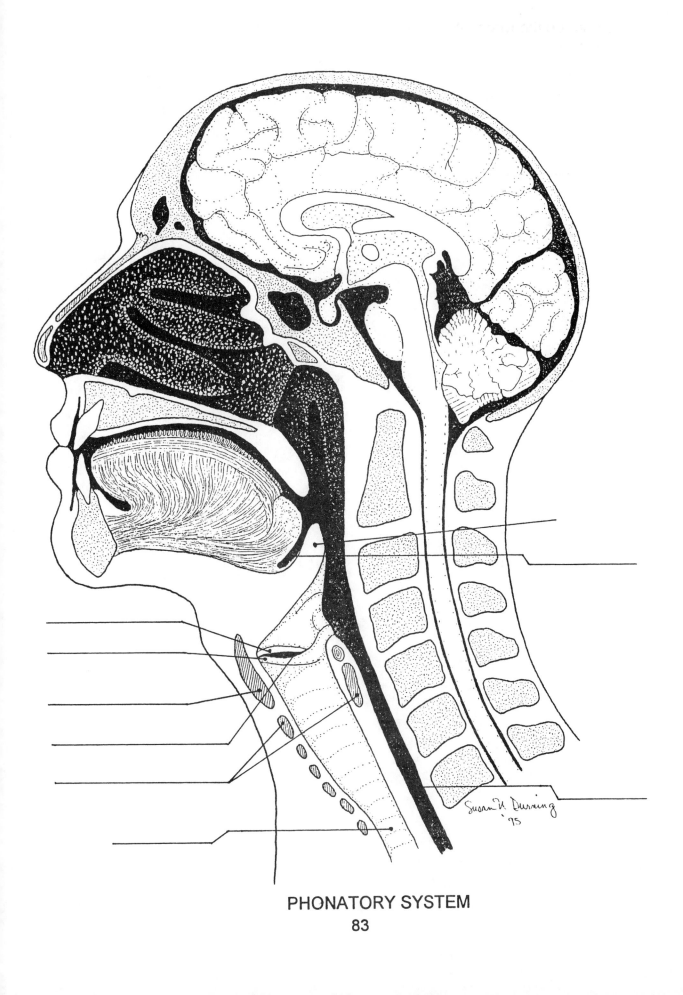

PHONATORY SYSTEM

83

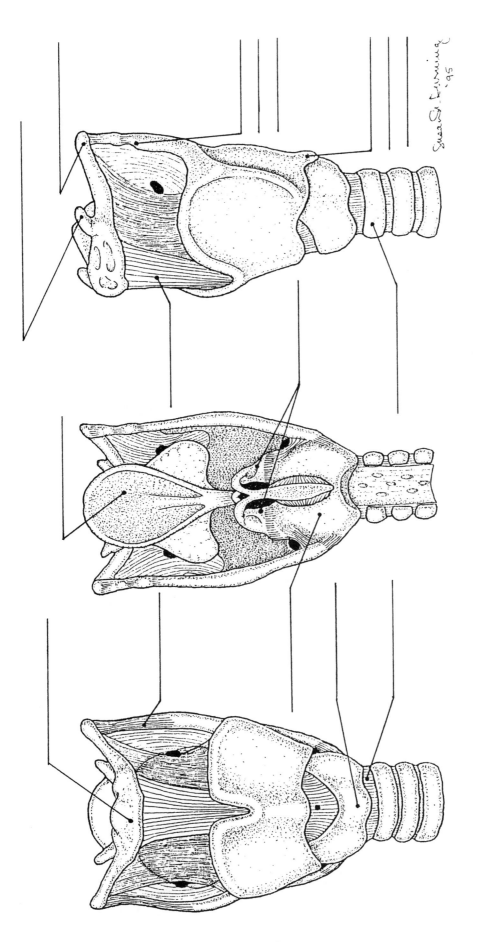

SKELETON OF THE LARYNX

85

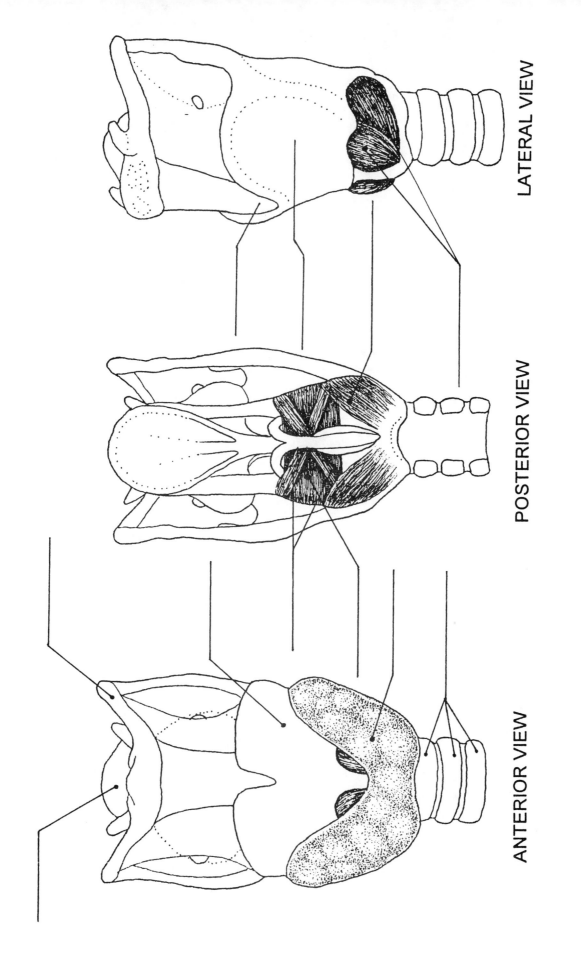

LATERAL VIEW

POSTERIOR VIEW

ANTERIOR VIEW

LARYNX

87

UNIT 5
THE ARTICULATORY MECHANISM

Synopsis of the Articulatory Mechanism

The primary functions of the articulatory structures are **mastication** (chewing), **deglutition** (swallowing), and **adjustment** of the opening of the airway. The overlaid function of speech production is the result of millions of years of evolution. Human beings discovered that the extreme flexibility of their **branchial** musculature enabled them to produce a broad array of sounds when they moved in relationship to the less mobile structures of the upper airway.

To produce speech, the compressed air stream from the lungs, either voiced or unvoiced, is shaped by the muscles and structures of articulation. Sounds produced this way are called **egressive**. Some languages employ sounds created by reversing the flow of air, filling the lungs during speech, with the resulting sounds termed **ingressive**.

Speech is articulated through alteration of the shape of the **vocal tract**. The vocal tract is essentially a tube. It extends from the **glottis** to the openings of the nose and mouth. The structures that are used to alter vocal tract shape are referred to collectively as **articulators**.

Typically, the articulators are divided into fixed and mobile structures. The mobile structures move in relationship to the fixed ones, restricting air or altering the resonating characteristics of the tube of the vocal tract.

The **fixed articulators** are the **upper incisors**, (superior) **alveolar ridge**, and the **hard palate**. The **upper incisors**, in combination with the tongue or lower lip, serve to create high frequency consonants. The **hard palate**, formed by the maxillae and the palatine bones, separates the nasal and oral cavities. The anterior portion of the hard palate, from which the upper incisors erupt, is the **superior alveolar ridge**. This portion of the maxilla is so important to speech that it is usually considered a separate articulator. Since the inferior alveolar ridge is not used for standard speech articulation, the anatomical locator term is usually dropped. The fixed articulators provide a surface against which to juxtapose the tongue or lips for the alteration of resonance and the modification of airflow.

The mobile articulators are the **lips, mandible, velum, tongue, pharyngeal walls** and **larynx**. The **lips** form a sphincter at the oral opening. They can occlude the oral cavity, articulate with the teeth, or form a ring through selective contraction of the **orbicularis oris** muscle. The formation of a labial ring serves as a fricative source or changes the resonance of the tract by extending its length and circular dimension. The **mandible** is mobile and adjusts oral cavity opening by elevating and depressing. It works synergistically with the **tongue** to produce the fine adjustments necessary for vowel productions. The tongue is the most important structure of speech articulation. It is a flexible muscular structure covered with mucous membrane. Tongue muscles are divided into **extrinsic** and **intrinsic** groups. Extrinsic muscles have one connection outside the tongue and they are further divided into suprahyoid and infra hyoid groups. Intrinsic muscles have both origin and attachment within the tongue. They are primarily involved in shaping the tongue for movement of food and liquid. They are also play an important role making the fine adjustments necessary for vowel and consonant productions. The **velum** extends posteriorly from the hard palate is continuous with it. It is a movable muscle that serves to couple or uncouple the nasal cavity with the rest of the vocal tract. It is closed during sucking and mastication.

The structures and muscles of articulation produce vowels and consonants of language phonology. These may be described by the amount or **manner** and location or **place** of maximum vocal tract constriction associated with their formations.   A third descriptor is the presence or absence of **voicing**. While all vowels are voiced, some consonants are not. Dynamic patterns of articulator movement, opening and closing the vocal tract in various manners and at various locations, produce the audible **syllables** of speech. The study of speech sounds is **phonetics**. Speech sounds may either form the nucleus of syllables or form syllable boundaries.

UNIT 5: THE ARTICULATORY MECHANISM
Objectives and Study Guide

Accomplishment of the objectives of this unit should provide the student with a basis for understanding the structure and function of the orofacial mechanism and the oropharynx. Checking the boxes beside each goal will help the student mark progress toward that understanding.

✐❒ 1. Describe the general anatomy of the vocal tract.

✐❒ 2. Describe the functions of the structures of the vocal tract in speech and swallowing.

✐❒ 3. Name the bones of the skull.

✐❒ 4. Describe the major divisions of the bones of the skull.

✐❒ 5. Name the structures of speech articulation.

✐❒ 6. Differentiate between the fixed and the mobile speech articulators.

✐❒ 7. Identify the cavities of the vocal tract and name the structures in each that are essential to normal speech and swallowing.

✐❒ 8. Name the muscles of facial expression essential to speech articulation.

✐❒ 9. Name the oral and pharyngeal muscles essential to normal speech and swallowing.

✐❒ 10. Describe, in general, the changes associated with normal growth of the head.

✐❒ 11. Describe the stages of deglutition.

UNIT 5: THE ARTICULATORY MECHANISM
Study Outline

I.   General Structure and Function of the Vocal Tract.

    A.   Structure
        Describe the locations of the following structures of the articulatory mechanism.
        1.   Oral Cavity

                a.   Tongue

                b.   Dental Arches

                c.   Hard Palate

                d.   Soft Palate

        2.   Nasal Cavity

                a.   Nares

                b.   Choanae

                c.   Septum

3.   Pharyngeal Cavity

    a.   Laryngopharynx

    b.   Oropharynx

    c.   Nasopharynx

II.   Function
Describe these functional aspects of the articulatory mechanism as they apply to speech and deglutition.

A.   Plosive and Fricative Sources for Obstruent Consonants
How do the structures of the oral cavity function to create constrictions for these sources? Are all obstruent consonants formed by constriction in the oral cavity?

B.   Analogy to Band-Pass Filter for Vowels and Semivowels
How do the muscles of the articulatory mechanism modify the phonatory source?

C.   General Function
Describe the oral cavity as the entrance to the alimentary canal.

III.   The Skull in General
        Describe these structures in the spaces provided.
        A.   Gross Structure
              1.   Skull

                    a.   Cranium

                          (1)   Facial Skeleton

                          (2)   Calvaria

                    b.   Mandible

                    c.   Hyoid bone

              2.   Cavities of the Cranium
                    Describe the locations and contents of these cavities of the cranium.

                    a.   Cranial Cavity

                    b.   Orbits

                    c.   Nasal Cavity

        B.   Bone Type

        C.   Mechanical Stresses

IV.   Superior Aspect of the Cranium

    A.   Calvaria
    What portion of the skull comprises the calvaria? Describe the locations of the following bones of the calvaria.

        1.   Frontal Bone

        2.   Temporal and Sphenoid Bones

        3.   Parietal Bones

        4.   Occipital Bone

    B.   Sutures
    What type of joint is a suture? How do these joints change as the individual develops? Describe the locations of the following sutures.

1.	Sagittal		4.	Pterion
2.	Coronal		5.	Lambda
3.	Lambda		6.	Bregma

V. Inferior Aspect of the Cranium
Describe the forms and locations of the following structures in the spaces provided.
A. Anterior Section

1. Hard Palate
Describe the functions of the hard palate in speech and in deglutition.

a. Maxilla

(1) Superior Alveolar Process

(2) Incisive Fossa

b. Palatine Bone

c. Superior Teeth
Identify the following teeth. Which teeth are essential for articulation of dental phonemes? Draw and label the superior dental arch of an adult in the box below.

(1) Incisors

(a) Central

(b) Lateral

(2) Cuspids

(3) Bicuspids

(4) Molars

2. Growth and Development of Teeth
By what age should the teeth necessary for the articulation of dental consonants erupt?

a. Teeth Eruption
Give the normal ages of eruption of the superior dentition.

b. Anomalies of Occlusion
Define the following terms for dental occlusion anomalies.
(1) Axiversion

    (a) Distoversion

    (b) Mesioversion

(2) Infraversion

(3) Supraversion

(4) Torsiversion

B.   Middle Section of the Skull
     Describe the sphenoid and occipital bones as structures of the middle, inferior aspect of the skull.

     1.   Nasopharynx
          Locate the nasopharynx with respect to the inferior aspect of the skull.

     2.   Sphenoid Bone
          a.   Pterygoid Plates
               Describe the pterygoid plates of the sphenoid bone as points of attachment for pharyngeal muscles.

               (1)   Pterygoid muscles
                     Describe the mandibular movement associated with these muscles. Why is this movement important in mastication?

               (2)   Tensor Veli Palatini
                     Describe the origins of this muscle. What role does it play in speech? Describe the hamular processes *of the sphenoid bone.*

3. Occipital Bone
What portion of the occipital bone contributes to speech articulation?

C. Posterior Section of the Inferior Skull

1. Occipital Bone
Describe the form and function of the following landmarks of the occipital bone in the spaces provided.
   a. Foramen Magnum

   b. Occipital Condyles

   c. Jugular Foramina

      (1) Internal Jugular Veins

      (2) Glossopharyngeal Nerves

      (3) Vagus Nerves

      (4) Accessory Nerves

   d. Carotid Canals

      (1) Internal Carotid Arteries

      (2) Sympathetic Plexuses

   e. Hypoglossal Canals

2. Temporal Bones
Describe the forms and functions of these landmarks of the temporal bones in the spaces provided.

a. Squamous Portions

b. Petrous Portions

(1) Auditory Meatuses

(2) Bony Labyrinths

c. Mastoid Processes
What muscles attach bilaterally to the sternum, clavicle, and the mastoid process?

d. Styloid Processes
What muscles attach to the styloid processes bilaterally?

VI. Anterior Aspect of the Skull
Describe the forms and functions of the structures of the anterior skull in the spaces provided.

A. The Face

1. Importance in Communication

a. Speech
Which facial structures are involved in speech?

b. Facial Expression
Of what importance is facial expression in communication?

2. Bones of the Face
Describe the locations of these bones of the face.
a. Frontal Bones

b. Maxillae

c. Zygomatic Bones

d. Nasal Bones

3. Landmarks of the Face
    *Write the locations of these facial landmarks in the spaces
    provided.*

    a. Frontal Eminences

    b. Orbits

    c. Nose

        (1) Nares

        (2) Nasal Septum

    d. Philtrum

VII. Lateral Aspect of the Skull
Describe these bones articulations and landmarks of the lateral aspect of the skull.
A.   Bones
1.   Frontal Bone

2.   Parietal Bone

3.   Sphenoid Bone

4.   Temporal Bone

a.   External Auditory Meatus

b.   Mastiod Process

c.   Styloid Process

5.   Occipital Bone

B.   Articulations
Describe the locations of the following articulations of the skull bones. Include the names of the bones involved.
1.   Temporo-Zygomatic

2.   Pterion

VIII. The Mandible
Describe these features of the mandible. Of what importance is the mandibular movement to normal speech?

   A.   Importance in Speech

         1.   Tongue Elevation

         2.   Opening of the Oral Cavity

         3.   Point of Attachment for Muscles of Speech Articulation
              Identify the muscles of speech articulation that attach directly to the mandible.

   B.   Importance in Deglutition
        Describe the importance of the mandible to mastication.

         1.   Opening of the Oral Cavity

         2.   Mastication
              Which muscles of mastication attach directly to the mandible?

C. Structure of the Mandible
    Describe the structure of the mandible in the spaces below.
    1. Corpus

        a. Mental Symphysis and Protuberance

        b. Inferior Alveolar Arch
            Of what importance are the mandibular teeth to speech?

    2. Ramus

        a. Condylar Process

        b. Temporomandibular Joint
            *Describe the origins and insertions of the muscles that
            elevate the mandible. Which muscles depress the
            mandible? When are they used?*

            (1) Muscles of Mandibular Elevation

            (2) Muscles of Mandibular Rotation

        c. Coronoid Process
            What muscle attaches to the coronoid process?

        d. Angle of the Mandible
            *How does the angle of the mandible change as the
            individual develops?*

IX.   The Speech Articulators
       A.   Overview
             1.   Form
                   Describe the structures and locations of the fixed and mobile speech articulators. State their roles in the production of specific obstruent consonants.

                   a.   Fixed Articulators

                         (1)   Upper Incisors

                         (2)   Superior Alveolar Ridge

                         (3)   Hard Palate (Maxillae)

                   b.   Mobile Articulators

                         (1)   Lips

                         (2)   Mandible

                         (3)   Soft Palate (Velum)

                         (4)   Tongue

                         (5)   Pharyngeal Walls

                         (6)   Larynx

             2.   Function in Speech
                   Describe how the speech articulators perform the following functions in the production of phonemes. Review place and manner of phoneme articulation.

                   a.   Modulation of Airflow for Consonant Articulation

                   b.   Alteration of Resonance for Vowel and Semivowel Articulation

3. Function in Deglutition
    Describe how the orofacial muscles perform the following functions in the intake of food and liquid.

    a.   Retention of Material in Oral Cavity

    b.   Sealing of Oral Cavity for Pressure Change

    c.   Mastication

    d.   Transfer of Bolus

    e.   Protection of Airway

B.	Oral Speech Articulators in Detail
	Describe these details of the oral speech articulators in the spaces provided.
	1.	Extraoral Articulators
		a.	Lips

			(1)	Vermillion Zone

			(2)	"Cupid's Bow"

			(3)	Effects of Lip Rounding

		b.	Muscles of Facial Expression
			Describe the origins and insertions of these muscles. Describe the effects of their contraction.
			(1)	Sphincteric Muscles

				(a)	Orbicularis Oris

				(b)	Orbicularis Oculi

			(2)	Horizontal Muscles

				(a)	Buccinator

				(b)	Risorus

			(3)	Angular Muscles

				(a)	Levator Labii Superiorus

				(b)	Levator Labii Superiorus Alaeque Nasi

				(c)	Zygomaticus Major

				(d)	Zygomaticus Minor

				(e)	Depressor Labii Inferiorus

(4) Vertical Muscles

    (a) Mentalis

    (b) Depressor Anguli Oris

    (c) Levator Anguli Oris

(5) Parallel Muscles

    (a) Incisivus Labi Superiorus

    (b) Incisivus Labi Inferiorus

Draw lines representing the courses of the fibers of the muscles of facial expression in the box below. Indicate the names of the muscles you are representing.

c.   Function of Extraoral Articulators

    (1)   Labial Consonants
        List the labial consonants using the International Phonetic Alphabet.

    (2)   Rounded Vowels
        List the rounded vowels of American English. Is lip rounding associated with articulation of any consonants?

    (3)   Gestural Communication

    (4)   Retention of Fluids

d.   Motor Innervation
What is the major peripheral nerve through which motor innervation of these muscles is provided?

e.   Sensory Innervation
Through which major peripheral nerve are sensations of pain, temperature and touch conveyed to the central nervous system?

2. Intraoral Articulators
Describe the form and functions of the following intraoral structures. What are their roles in the articulation of speech?
a. Roof of the Oral Cavity
What are the possible effects of an unrepaired fistula (cleft) of the roof of the oral cavity?

   (1) Maxilla (Hard Palate)

      (a) Tissue Type

      (b) Superior Alveolar Ridge

      (c) Upper Dental Arch

   (2) Velum (Soft Palate)

      (a) Uvula

      (b) Velopharyngeal Sphincter

         i) Muscles of the Velopharyngeal Sphincter

            a) Tensor Veli Palatini

            b) Levator Veli Palatini

            c) Palatopharyngeus

            d) Palatoglossus

ii)   Function of the Velopharyngeal
        Sphincter

iii)   Motor Innervation
        *Which peripheral nerves convey
        motor impulses from the central
        nervous system to the
        velopharyngeal sphincter muscles?*

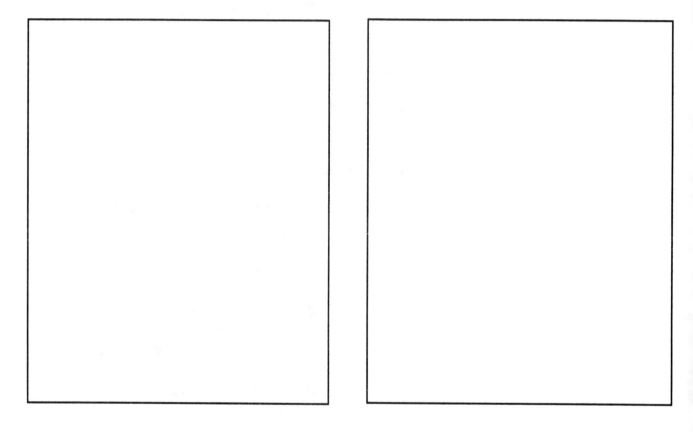

*Draw a schematic representation
of a mid sagittal view of the oral
cavity in the box above. Include
the lips, tongue, upper teeth and
the velum.*

*Draw a schematic representation
of the open oral cavity as seen
from the anterior aspect. Include
the lips, tongue, upper teeth and
the velum.*

b.   Floor of the Oral Cavity

    (1)   The Tongue
    Describe the role of the tongue in the articulation of speech. List the consonants produced by articulation of the tongue with the other oral structures. Describe the role of the tongue in the articulation of vowels.

        (a)   Gross Structure of the Tongue

            i)   Parts of the Tongue
                a)   Apex
                b)   Dorsum
                c)   Blade
                d)   Root

            ii)   Tissue Type of the Tongue

            iii)   Landmarks of the Tongue

            iv)   Attachments of the Tongue

            v)   Intrinsic Muscles of the Tongue

                a)   Vertical

                b)   Transverse

                c)   Superior Longitudinal

                d)   Inferior Longitudinal

vi)   Extrinsic Muscles of the Tongue

    a)   Genioglossus

    b)   Styloglossus

    c)   Hyoglossus

    d)   Palatoglossus

vii)   Motor Innervation of the Tongue

viii)   Sensory Innervation of the Tongue
What is the role of the touch and stretch receptors of the tongue in the treatment of articulatory disorders? Do taste receptors have a role in the treatment of swallowing disorders?

    a)   Touch

    b)   Taste

c.   Posterior Oral Cavity

  (1)   Faucial Pillars

    (a)   Palatoglossus

    (b)   Palatopharyngeus

    (c)   Tonsillar Fossa

(2)   Tonsils (Waldeyer's Ring)

     (a)   Palatine

     (b)   Pharyngeal (Adenoid)

     (c)   Lingual

     (d)   Functions

     (e)   Relevance to Speech Pathology

(3)   Posterior (Oro-) Pharyngeal Wall
What functions do the posterior oral and pharyngeal structures have in modifying the quality of the speech signal?

     (a)   Superior and Middle Pharyngeal Constrictors

     (b)   Passavant's Pad

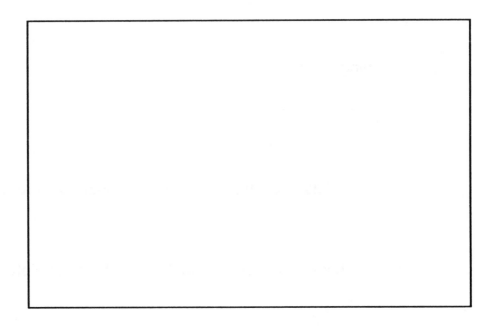

In the box above, draw a midsagittal view of the oral cavity. Show the tongue, hard palate and velum in the closed position.

X.   Deglutition

    A.   Three Stages of Deglutition
       Describe the progress of a bolus of food during each of these stages of deglutition

       1.   Oral Stage (Voluntary)

          a.   Preparation of the Bolus

          b.   Elevation of Oral Floor

          c.   Posterior Propulsion of Bolus

          d.   Constriction of Posterior Oral Cavity

          e.   Closing of Velopharyngeal Sphincter

       2.   Pharyngeal Stage (Involuntary)

          a.   Approximation of Aryepiglottic Folds

          b.   Arytenoid Cartilages Drawn Superiorly and Anteriorly

          c.   Elevation of Larynx and Articulation of Epiglottis

       3.   Esophageal Stage (Involuntary)

UNIT 5: THE ARTICULATORY MECHANISM
Self Test

1. Which part of the skull includes the calvarium and the facial skeleton?
   _____ & _____.

2. A person viewing the skull from the lateral aspect would see which bones?
   _____.

3. The cheeks are formed by which bones? _____.

4. The mental protuberance is part of which bone? _____.

5. What are the three cavities of the vocal tract? _____,
   _____ & _____.

6. Name the cavities of the cranium. _____.

7. The frontal bone forms which facial structure? _____.

8. Which muscles elevate the posterior part of the tongue? _____.

9. Which of the following are *mobile* articulators?

   a)Tongue; b)Teeth; c)Alveolar Ridge; d)Velum; e)Lips

10. A fistula between the oral and nasal cavities is commonly called a _____
    _____.

11. Which facial muscle(s) contract(s) when the speaker forms /u/? _____
    _____.

12. Which stage of deglutition is voluntary? _____.

13. Which muscles contract to elevate the mandible? _____
    _____.

14. Which articulators must function to produce /s/? _____.

15. Describe the changes to the angle of the mandible that are coincident with
    aging. _____
    _____
    _____.

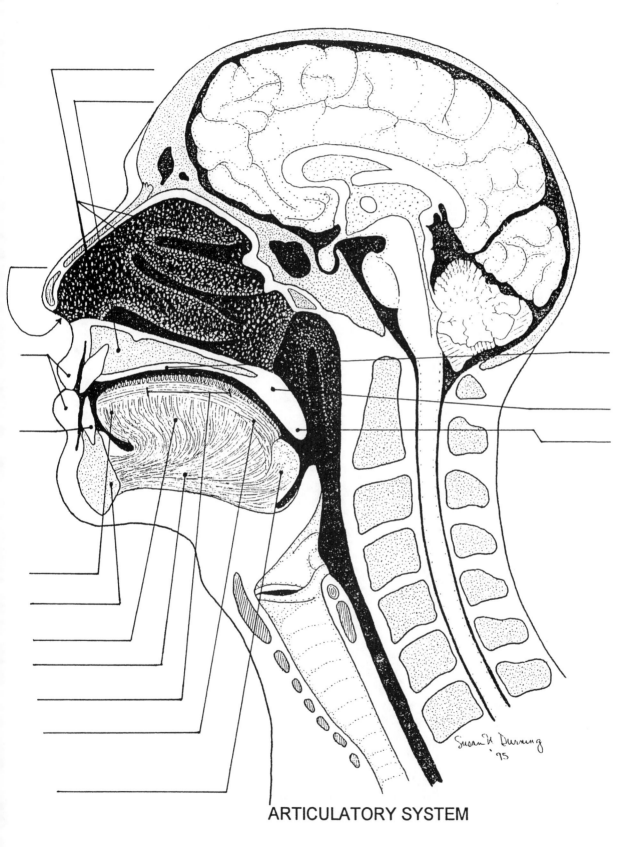

ARTICULATORY SYSTEM

121

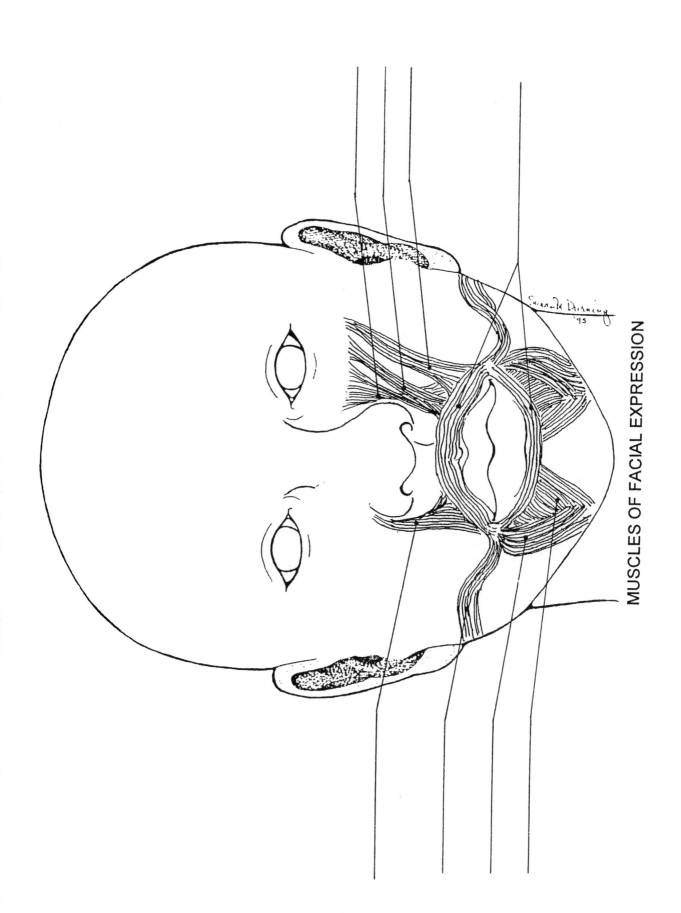

MUSCLES OF FACIAL EXPRESSION

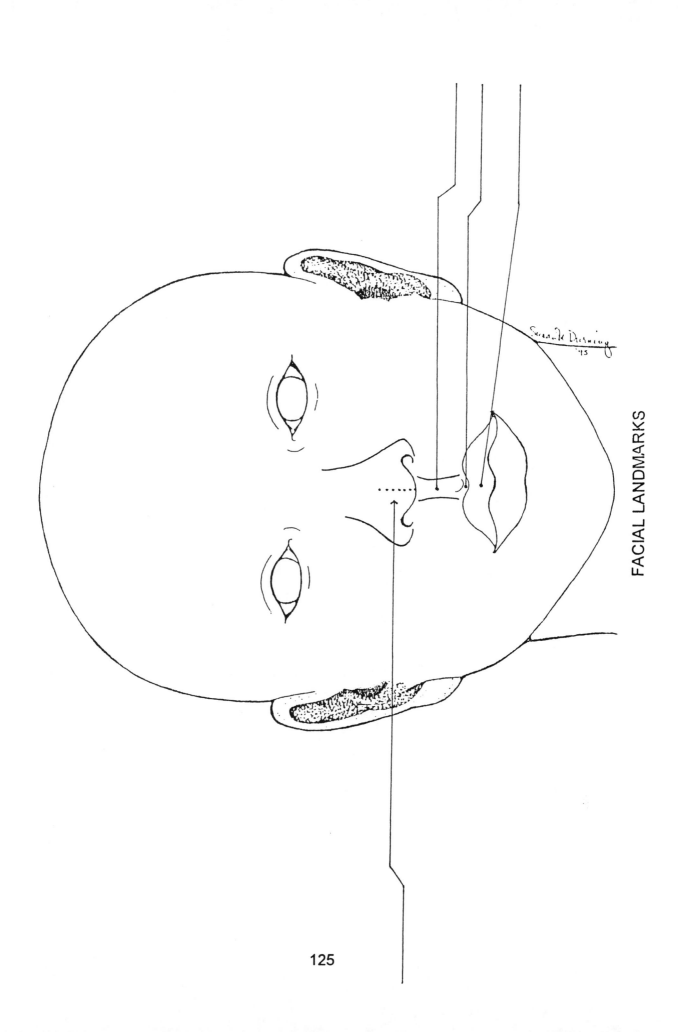

FACIAL LANDMARKS

125

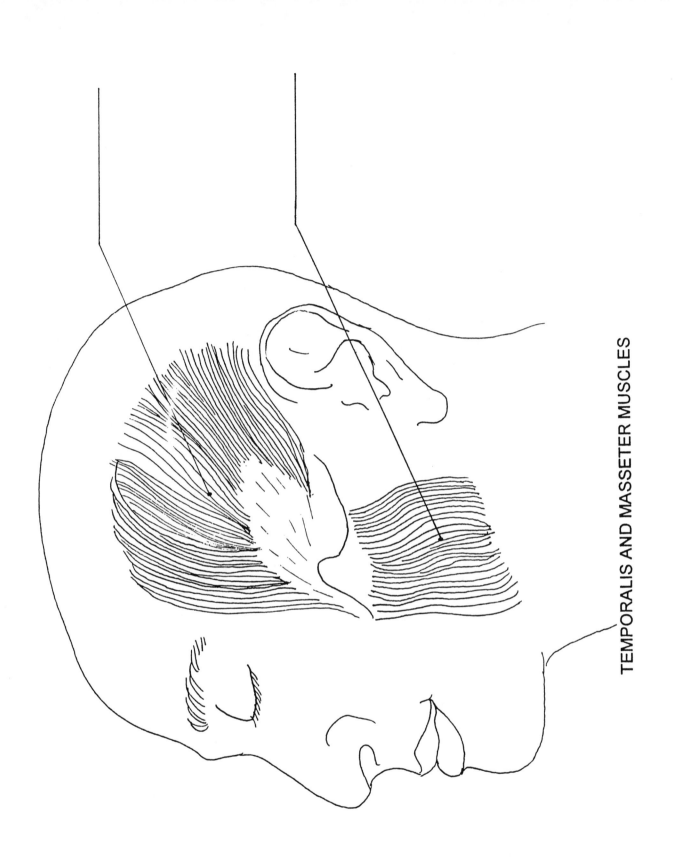

TEMPORALIS AND MASSETER MUSCLES

127

UNIT 6
THE NERVOUS SYSTEM

The nervous system is the medium by which the body realizes its wants and needs. Acting in concert with the endocrine system, the nervous system serves its function by virtue of the special conductivity and directionality of its constituent nervous tissue. The basic structure of the nervous system consists of the functional **neuron** and supportive **glial** tissues. The neuron consists of the **cell body** (soma), **axon, dendrite** and the **synaptic junction**. It propagates ionic changes, called action potentials or neural impulses. These changes travel from the dendrites, past the cell body, to the axon. From there, they cross the cleft of the synapse to the next dendrite.

Anatomists divide the nervous system into central and peripheral systems, but these divisions are for convenience only. The nervous system functions as a whole.

The central nervous system consists of the **brain** and **spinal cord**. Both are contained in the axial skeleton, and are covered by three membranes, the meninges. The central nervous system mediates input from the peripheral nerves and effects its responses through them.

The brain is divided into two **hemispheres** connected by the **corpus callosum**. It contains more than twenty billion nerve cells and exercises executive control over higher mental sensory and motor functions. **Motor** and **sensory** functions of the right hemisphere are responsible for voluntary control and sensation on the left side of the body and vice versa. A **dominant hemisphere**, usually the left hemisphere, performs the crucial role in the reception and expression of language.

The gray **cerebral cortex** is a thin layer of cells covering the surface of the brain. It is a **convoluted** structure with **gyri** (ridges) and **sulci** (valleys) that serve as major anatomical landmarks for anatomists. Major sulci of the cortex include the **lateral, central** and **lunate** sulci. The major gyri of the cerebral cortex include the **precentral, postcentral, angular, supramarginal gyri** and the **pars triangularis. Broca's** and **Wernicke's** areas are the major expressive and receptive speech and language centers, working in concert to perceive, formulate, express and monitor spoken language.

There are four **lobes** of the cerebrum named after the bones of the skull under which they are located: **frontal, parietal, temporal** and **occipital**. The neuronal tissue of all the cerebral lobes receive, relay, reverberate, store and retrieve impulses from external and internal sources. None functions as an independent unit. The personality of an individual is the result of the combined functioning of all parts of the nervous system. The frontal lobe is the largest and forms the anterior portion of the hemisphere. The **motor cortex** and Broca's area are located in the frontal lobe. The **Fissure of Rolando** or **central sulcus** divides the frontal and parietal lobes. The **primary motor cortex** lies immediately anteriorly to the central sulcus and the **primary sensory cortex** is posterior to this major landmark. The parietal lobe, forming the superior lateral portion of the hemisphere, is associated with the interpretation of sensory information. The **angular** and **supramarginal** gyri are also located in the parietal lobe. These gyri are associated with the interpretation of symbolic stimuli. The temporal lobe comprises the inferior lateral section of the hemisphere. It is associated with the interpretation of auditory input. The **auditory cortex** or **Heschl's Gyrus** is located in the temporal lobe. The **Fissure of Sylvius**, or **lateral sulcus**, separates the temporal and frontal lobes. At the posterior region of the brain, the occipital lobe is delineated by the **lunate sulci**, visible on the medial surfaces of the hemispheres. The **primary visual cortex** is found in the occipital lobe. The **insular cortex** is sometimes identified as a cerebral lobe. It is located deep to the lateral fissure and is only visible by separating the bordering cortical tissue.

The interior of the brain contains the **white matter** and is made up of **afferent** and **efferent projection** fibers. White fibers are so called because they are sheathed in a white fatty **myelin sheath**. They converge at the **internal capsules** and **thalami** of each hemisphere, and descend through the **midbrain, pons,** and **medulla** levels of the **brainstem**. The white matter also contains **commissural** and **association** fibers that connect centers within and between the cerebral hemispheres.

Four **ventricles**, cavities filled with **cerebrospinal** fluid, are deep within the white matter. Cerebrospinal fluid is created in these ventricles and flows out and around the central nervous system. The fluid protects the central nervous system and helps regulate intracranial pressure.

The circulation of blood is critical to brain function. Neuronal tissues die very shortly after interruption in their ability to perform metabolism. Central nervous system neurons have very limited regenerative ability and are generally replaced with structural **glial** tissue after they die. The **internal carotid** and **vertebral arteries** supply blood to the brain. They conjoin at the **Circle of Willis** where **anterior, posterior** and **middle** cerebral arteries provide the primary blood supply to the hemispheres. Venous drainage is provided by the **dural sinuses** and the **jugular veins**.

The **spinal cord** is the caudal extension of the brainstem. It is the major conduit for impulses passing to or from the central nervous system. The spinal cord, as a central nervous system structure, processes some reflexive neural information.

Spinal cord functions are said to be **segmental**.

The peripheral nervous system consists of the **twelve cranial nerves, thirty one spinal nerves,** and the **autonomic nervous system.** The cranial nerves have synaptic connections with the brainstem. They are final common pathways for most of the sensory and motor functions of the peripheral speech and hearing mechanisms. Spinal nerves synapse at nuclei at or very close to the spinal cord. The autonomic nervous system has both **sympathetic** and **parasympathetic** divisions that maintain and regulate unconscious bodily functions or adapt them in emergencies.

UNIT 6: THE NERVOUS SYSTEM
Objectives and Study Guide

The objectives for this unit are to provide the student a foundation upon which to base further study of this vastly complex subject. Students should mark progress by checking the boxes beside each objective as they accomplish them.

1. Describe the general organization of the human nervous system.

2. Differentiate between afferent and efferent nervous functions.

3. Describe the major components of the central nervous system.

4. Name the major parts of the human brain.

5. Name and describe the general functions of the lobes of the cerebral cortex.

6. Identify, using diagrams or models, the major landmarks of the cerebral cortex and associate their general functions.

7. Identify, using diagrams, the major subcortical structures of the brain and associate their major functions.

8. Identify and describe the general function of the cerebellum.

9. Name and describe the three meninges and their relative locations.

10. Describe the flow of cerebrospinal fluid.

11. Describe the major components of the peripheral nervous system.

12. Name and describe the communication functions of the cranial nerves.

13. Name and describe some commonly encountered syndromes associated with disorders of the human nervous system.

UNIT 6: THE NERVOUS SYSTEM
Study Outline

I.   General Organization of the Human Nervous System
        Describe the overall organization of the human nervous system. How do the two major divisions serve each other? Is it realistic to consider the system as comprised of two separate entities?

        A.   Basic Structure

                1.   The Neuron

                        a.   Cell Body

                        b.   Axon

                        c.   Dendrite

                        d.   Synapses

                2.   Glial Tissue

B. Central Nervous System
Describe the locations and general functions of the major parts of the central nervous system.
1. Brain

   a. Cerebral Hemispheres

      (1) Cerebral Cortex

         (a) Location

         (b) General Function

   b. Subcortical Structures

      (a) Location

      (b) General Function

   c. Brainstem

      (1) Location

      (2) General Function

   d. Cerebellum

      (1) Location

      (2) General Function

2.   Spinal Cord

    a.   Location

    b.   General Function

C.   Peripheral Nervous System

    1.   Spinal and Cranial Nerves
Give the general locations of the nuclei of the cranial and the spinal nerves. Describe the general differences in functions between the cranial nerves and the spinal nerves.

        a.   12 Cranial Nerves

        b.   31 Spinal Nerves

    2.   Autonomic Nervous System (Ganglia and Nerve Processes)
Describe the general differences between the sympathetic and parasympathetic divisions of the autonomic nervous system
        a.   Sympathetic Division

        b.   Parasympathetic Division

II. The Brain in Detail
Describe the form and functions of these structures of the brain.

A. Cerebral Hemispheres

1. Cerebral Cortex

a. Structure of the Cerebral Cortex

(1) Major Sulci of the Cerebral Cortex

(a) Lateral Sulcus (Fissure of Sylvius)

i) Location of the Lateral Sulcus

ii) Insula

iii) Opercula

iv) Parallel Sulcus

(b) Central Sulcus (Fissure of Rolando)

i) Location of the Central Sulcus

ii) Precentral and Postcentral Functions

(c) Lunate Sulcus (Simian Sulcus)

(2) Major Gyri of the Cerebral Cortex
Describe the locations of these gyri of the cerebral cortex.

    (a)   Precentral gyrus

    (b)   Postcentral Gyrus

    (c)   Angular Gyrus

    (d)   Supramarginal Gyrus

    (e)   Pars Triangularis

b.   General Functions of Areas of the Cerebral Cortex
Describe the locations of these specific areas of the cerebral cortex. Draw their locations in the space provided.

    (1)   Sensory Cortex

    (2)   Motor Cortex

    (3)   Auditory Cortex

    (4)   Visual Cortex

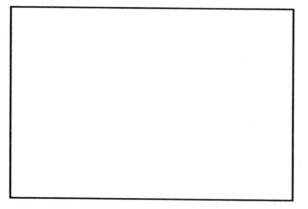

2.   Hemispheric Functions

   a.   Interhemispheric Differences

      (1)   Cerebral Dominance
            What is meant by "cerebral dominance?"

            (a)   Incidence of Left or Right Hemisphere
                  Dominance

            (b)   Relationship to Handedness

      (2)   Dominant Hemisphere Functions

      (3)   Non-Dominant Hemisphere Functions

   b.   Interhemispheric Communication
        *Name and locate the major interhemispheric
        connections.*

   c.   Intrahemispheric Communication
        *Name and locate the major intrahemispheric
        communication pathways.*

3. Lobes of the Cerebral Cortex
Describe the forms and functions of the following structures of the cerebral cortex.

    a.   Frontal Lobe

        (1)   Location

        (2)   Functions
                Describe and name the possible effects of a lesion in the following locations.

                (a)   Motor Cortex (Precentral Gyrus)

                        i)   Homunculus (Projections)

                        ii)   Decussation of Motor Tracts

                (b)   Association Areas

                        i)   Premotor Cortex

                        ii)   Broca's Area (Pars Triangularis)

                (c)   Other Functions

b.   Parietal Lobe

    (1)   Location

        (a)   Postcentral Gyrus

        (b)   Somesthetic Cortex (Sensory Cortex)

    (2)   Functions
Describe the possible effects of a lesion in the following locations.

        (a)   Sensory Decussation

        (b)   Sensory Homunculus

        (c)   Stereognosis
Define stereognosis. What role does stereognosis play in the production (or perception) of speech?

    (3)   Angular Gyrus
What effect might a lesion in this area have on communication?

    (4)   Supramarginal Gyrus
What effect might a lesion in this area have on communication?

c.   Temporal Lobe

    (1)   Location

        (a)   Temporal Gyri

        (b)   Auditory Cortex (Heschl's Gyri)

    (2)   Functions
Describe and name the possible effects of a temporal lobe lesion on the following functions.

        (a)   Sensation

        (b)   Perception

        (c)   Association

    (3)   Wernicke's Area

    (4)   Meyer's Loop

d.   Occipital Lobe

    (1)   Location

        (a)   Parieto-occipital Fissure

        (b)   Calcarine Sulcus

        (c)   Visual Cortex

    (2)   Functions
Describe and name the possible effects of a lesion on the following occipital lobe functions.

        (a)   Sensation

            i)   Retinal Projections

            ii)   Optic Decussation
What is a "decussation?" Be alert for other examples of decussation in the central nervous system.

            iii)   Anopsia

        (b)   Perception

        (c)   Association

4.   Subcortical Structures
Describe the locations and functions of these subcortical structures in the spaces provided. Indicate the structures for which researchers have yet to reveal clear roles. Describe the possible effects of lesions in the following areas.

   a.   Thalamus

        (1)   Location

        (2)   Structure

        (3)   Function

   b.   Hypothalamus

   c.   Pineal Body

   d.   Basal Ganglia (Striate Bodies)

        (1)   Names

        (2)   General Location

        (3)   Structure

        (4)   Functions
              What effect might a lesion in this area have on communication?

5. Brainstem
    Draw a schematic representation of the brainstem and label the three major divisions.
    a. Location

        (1) Midbrain

        (2) Pons

        (3) Medulla

    b. Relationship to Spinal Cord

    c. Functions
        Briefly describe these central nervous system functions aggregated in the brainstem.
        (1) Ascending/Descending Tracts (CNS)

            (a) Decussations

                i)   Motor

                    a) Pyramidal

                    b) Extrapyramidal

                ii) Sensory

                    a) Spinothalamic Tracts

                    b) Trigeminothalamic Tracts

            (b) Reticular System

            (c) Vestibular System

147

6. Cerebellum

    a. Location

    b. Function

7. Meninges

    a. Dura

    b. Arachnoid

    c. Pia

8. Cerebrospinal Fluid (CSF)

    a. Composition

    b. Ventricles

    c. Foramina

    d. Subarachnoid Space

    e. Flow of Cerebrospinal Fluid
        Describe the production, flow and absorption of cerebrospinal fluid in the space below.

III.   Peripheral Nervous System

    1.   Spinal and Cranial Nerves
    Describe the differences in functions between the cranial nerves and the spinal nerves.

        a.   12 Cranial Nerves
        Beside each cranial nerve name, write its communicative function(s). Use the letters "S," "M," OR "B" to indicate if the nerve has "sensory," "motor," or "both" functions.

            (1)   I   Olfactory

            (2)   II   Optic

            (3)   III   Oculomotor

            (4)   IV   Trochlear

            (5)   V   Trigeminal

            (6)   VI   Abducens

            (7)   VII   Facial

            (8)   VIII   Vestibulocochlear

            (9)   IX   Glossopharyngeal

            (10)   X   Vagus

            (11)   XI   Accessory

            (12)   XII   Hypoglossal

        b.   31 Spinal Nerves
        Where are the spinal nerves located? What communicative functions do the spinal nerves have?

2. Autonomic Nervous System (Ganglia and Nerve Processes)
   Describe the general differences between the sympathetic and parasympathetic divisions of the autonomic nervous system

   a. Sympathetic

      (1) Thoracolumbar Outflow

      (2) Emergency Actions

   b. Parasympathetic

      (1) Craniosacral Outflow

      (2) Normal Bodily Functions

UNIT 6: THE NERVOUS SYSTEM
Self Test

1.   What are the two main divisions of the human nervous system?
     _____ & _____.

2.   The central nervous system is composed of _____ & _____.

3.   Sensory input is carried over _____ tracts.

4.   Motor impulses are carried over _____ tracts.

5.   The primary motor cortex is located in the _____ lobe.

6.   There are _____ pairs of cranial nerves.

7.   The spinal nerves are parts of the _____ nervous system.

8.   The peripheral nervous system is subdivided into which parts? _____
     _____.

9.   The emergency acceleration in heart rate and increased perspiration which accompanies the presence of anxiety evoking stimuli is accomplished through action of:_____.

10. The recognition that the (above) anxiety evoking stimuli are present is mediated by_____.

11. Nerves connect to one another at _____.

12. The raised portions of the convoluted surface of the cerebral hemispheres are called_____.

13. The temporal lobe is separated from the parietal and frontal lobes by _____.

14. The precentral and postcentral gyri are separated by_____
     _____.

15. The gyrus immediately posterior to the central sulcus is attributed with the function of_____.

16. Broca's area is located in the_____.

17. What condition will result when the visual cortex of one cerebral hemisphere is destroyed?_____.

18. A unilateral lesion of the motor cortex of the right hemisphere will result in _____.

19. The midbrain, pons, and medulla are parts of the_____.

20. The intrinsic muscles of the tongue receive their motor innervation via which cranial nerve? _____.

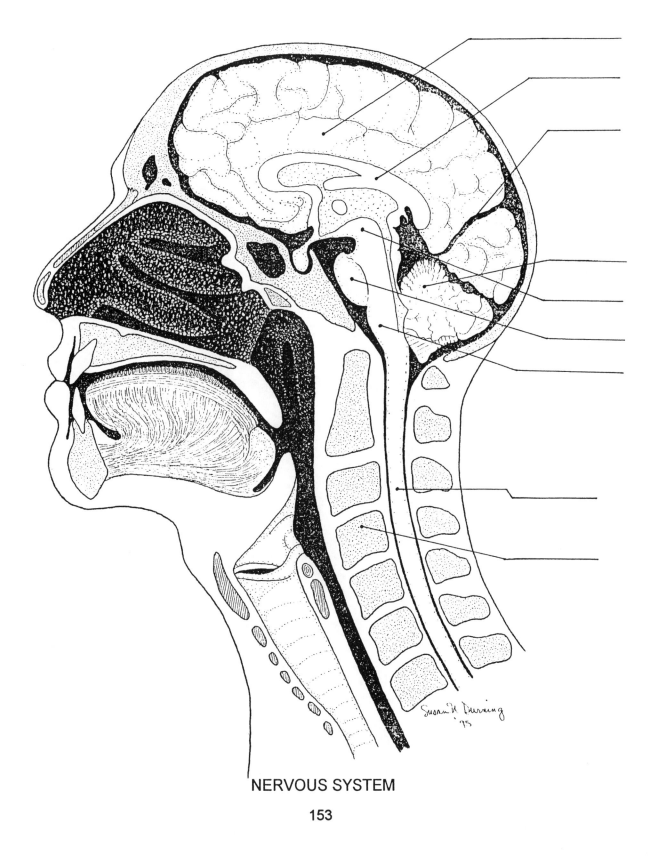

NERVOUS SYSTEM

UNIT 7
THE AUDITORY SYSTEM

Synopsis of the Auditory System

The process of hearing depends on the transmission and transformation of energy. **Acoustic** energy must pass through three media and be converted into the **electrochemical** energy of the nervous system before the listener becomes aware of its presence. The clarity with which the sound will be heard will depend upon the successful transmission of vibration energy from air to body tissues, and then to fluid.

Sound begins as the disruption of random molecular movements in a **medium**, usually air, by the directed displacements of a vibrating body. The vibrating body is referred to as the **source**.

Molecules in all matter are simultaneously attracted to and repelled from one another by the atomic forces of their components. The source applies additional force to adjacent molecules, and a chain reaction begins. Thus, the sound is **propagated**. Each displaced molecule in the medium absorbs some of the energy exerted upon it, but passes the residual energy on to the ones nearby. The process by which the molecules approach each other and bounce back is known as **compression** and **rarefaction**. Compression occurs when the distance between molecules is decreased and rarefaction occurs when the distance between the molecules is greater than during the normal state.

The listener becomes aware of the presence of sound when air molecules near the ear are set into motion with characteristics resembling those of the source. The sound must be of sufficient strength, or **intensity**, and within the anatomically determined range of **frequencies** to be transmitted by the ear and detected by the brain.

The **pinna** channels acoustic energy into the middle ear. The **external auditory meatus**, in its normal anatomical form, enhances sounds within the acoustic range of speech, and protects the sensitive deep structures of the auditory system. The external meatus leads to the **tympanic membrane**. The tympanic membrane divides the **outer** and **middle ear** and vibrates at a frequency and amplitude corresponding to the molecular displacements in the external meatus.

Sound energy passes on to the **middle ear**, or **tympanum**. The middle ear is an aspirin-sized cavity in the temporal bones of the skull. Since the cavity is closed at each end, a **eustachian tube** passes from within to the nasopharynx. This tube serves to equalize air pressure when required. Secured to the tympanic membrane are the three tiny bones of the middle ear known as the **ossicles: malleus, incus** and **stapes**. These bones vibrate in unison with the tympanic membrane and amplify the energy transmitted to the inner ear.

157

The **inner ear** contains the sensory end organ of hearing, the **cochlea**. The cochlea is part of a complex sensory structure called the **labyrinth**. The labyrinth is so named because it consists of soft tissue organs embedded in a series of tunnels hollowed out of the temporal bone of the skull. The cochlear tunnel is snail-shaped. Here, the medium of sound transmission becomes a fluid called **endolymph**. The fluid within the cochlea is set into vibration, which in turn, sets the **organ of corti** on the **basilar membrane** into vibration. This vibration occurs at a frequency and amplitude corresponding to the ossicular chain vibration. Attached to the organ of corti are epithelial **hair cells**, connected to the nerve endings of the **spiral ganglion**. Each hair cell movement sets off a subsequent neurological impulse along the **vestibulocochlear** or **eighth cranial nerve**. At this stage of the hearing process, the hydraulic energy occurring in the cochlea transforms into nerve or electrochemical energy.

The vestibulocochlear nerve enters the brainstem at a structure called the **medulla**. From the medulla, some nerve fibers enter a structure known as the **thalamus**. It is the thalamus, in combination with other brain structures, that regulates which auditory signals are attend to and those to be ignored. From the thalamus, the electrochemical energy is transmitted upward to the cortex where interpretation of the sound occurs.

Another sensory structure of the labyrinth is the **vestibular system**. This system senses the pull of gravity on its receptors. Its nerve endings interact with the body's axial and appendicular skeletal muscles, and with the extraocular eye muscles. The vestibular system helps the body maintain its posture through the sense of balance. It consists of the **utricle**, the **saccule** and three **semicircular canals**.

UNIT 7: THE AUDITORY SYSTEM
Objectives and Study Guide

Objectives for this unit are intended to orient the student to the fundamental form and function of the auditory system. With such preparation, the student should be ready to pursue further study in either audiology, speech-language pathology, or related fields. Students should check the boxes beside each objective to mark progress toward that overall goal.

1. Identify and describe the functions of the two main divisions of the human auditory system.

2. Describe the structures of the human auditory system as being located in the peripheral or central divisions of the auditory system.

3. Identify the anatomical limits and describe the functions of the peripheral hearing mechanism.

4. Name the three main parts of the peripheral hearing mechanism.

5. Describe the structures of the peripheral hearing mechanism as being located in the external, middle or inner ear(s).

6. Locate the major landmarks of the pinna.

7. Name and describe the morphologies and locations of the ossicles.

8. Describe the major functions of the parts of the peripheral hearing mechanism, including:

The Pinna
The External Auditory Meatus
The Tympanic Membrane
The Tympanum
The Eustachian Tubes

The Ossicles
The Cochlea
The Vestibule
The Semicircular Canals
The Vestibulocochlear Nerve

✏️☐ 9.   Identify and describe the functions of the following structures of the cochlea:

Scala Media   Organ of Corti
Scala Tympani   Hair Cells
Scala Vestibuli   Reissner's Membrane
Basilar Membrane   Endolymph
Tectorial Membrane   Perilymph
Auditory Nerve   Helicotrema

✏️☐ 10. Identify the anatomical limits and describe the functions of the central auditory system.

✏️☐ 11. Describe, in sequence, the transmission of auditory evoked potentials with respect to the following central auditory system structures:

Cochlear Nuclei
Superior Olivary Complex
Medial Geniculate Body of the Thalamus
Cerebral Cortex

UNIT 7: THE AUDITORY SYSTEM
Study Outline

I. Two Main Divisions of the Human Auditory System
Describe the location and functions of the two main divisions of the human auditory system.

    A. Peripheral Auditory System

        1. Location and Extent

        2. Functions

    B. Central Auditory System

        1. Location and Extent

        2. Functions

II. The Peripheral Hearing Mechanism in Detail
Describe the forms (extent) and functions of the following structures of the peripheral hearing mechanism in the spaces provided.

A. External (Outer) Ear

1. Pinna (Auricle)

a. Form
Locate the following parts of the pinna and label them on the accompanying illustration.
(1) Helix
(2) Antihelix
(3) Tragus
(4) Antitragus
(5) Lobe
(6) Concha
(7) Triangular Fossa

b. Functions of the Pinna
What are the hearing functions of the pinna? Does the pinna have functions other than those for hearing?

2. External Auditory Meatus

a. Form

(1) Ear Canal

(a) Shape

(b) Underlying Tissue Composition

(c) Cerumen
What are the origin and purposes of cerumen?

(2) Tympanic Membrane
Is the tympanic membrane part of the outer or middle ear? in the

   (a)   Laminae

   (b)   Pars Tensa

   (c)   Pars Flaccida

   (d)   Otoscopic Landmarks
Draw a schematic rep[resentation of the tympanic membrane as seen from the external auditory meatus in the box above. Label the following landmarks.

   i)   Pars Tensa

   ii)   Pars Flaccida

   iii)   Malleolar Stria

b.   Functions
Describe the functions of the external ear in the spaces provided.
(1)   Acoustic Function

(2)   Protective Function

c.   Mastoid Process (of Temporal bone)
How do audiologists use the mastoid process to specify the natures of hearing disorders?

163

B. Middle Ear (Tympanum)
    Describe these aspects of the middle ear in the spaces provided.

    1. General Form and Extent

    2. Function

    3. Structures of the Middle Ear

        a. Tympanic Membrane

            (1) Structure
                 Describe the laminae of the tympanic membrane.

            (2) Function

        b. Ossicles

            (1) Form
                 In the box on the right, draw a stylized diagram of the relationship of the ossicular chain to the tympanic membrane and to the oval window. Label each ossicle.

                 (a) Malleus

                 (b) Incus

                 (c) Stapes

(2)   Impedance Matching Function
Describe two ways the ossicular chain matches acoustic impedance between the atmosphere and the cochlear fluids.

c.   Eustachian (Pharyngotympanic) Tubes

(1)   Structure and Location

(2)   Function

d.   Muscles of the Middle Ear

(1)   Stapedius

(2)   Tensor Tympani

(3)   Acoustic Reflex
Does the acoustic reflex serve a protective function?

4.   Middle Ear Function Testing
Describe how audiologists test the function of the middle ear. Why is the otoscope an important tool in the examination of the peripheral hearing mechanism?

C.   Inner Ear (Labyrinth)

    1.   Location
        In what portion of the temporal bone is the inner ear located?

    2.   Bony Labyrinth

    3.   Membranous Labyrinth

    4.   Inner Ear Structures

        a.   Hearing Mechanism

            (1)   Cochlea

                (a)   Shape
                      Describe the shape of the cochlea. How many turns does it make from basal to apical ends?

                      i)   Basal End

                      ii)   Apical End

                (b)   Membranous Portion of the Cochlea

                      i)   Scala Media
                          Where are these fluids found relative to the scala media?

                          a)   Endolymph

                          b)   Perilymph

ii) Basilar Membrane
Describe these structures of the basilar membrane.
   a) Organ of Corti

   b) Hair Cells

   c) Tectorial Membrane

   d) Spiral Ganglion

iii) Reissner's (Vestibular) Membrane

(c) Bony Portion of the Cochlea
Describe the locations of these structures of the bony portion of the cochlea. What hearing function do these structures play?
   i) Scala Tympani

   ii) Scala Vestibuli

   iii) Helicotrema

   iv) Modiolus

(2) Cochlear Nerve
What is the other division of the eighth cranial nerve?

   i) VIIIth Cranial Nerve: Auditory Division

   ii) Cochlear Nerve Nuclei

   iii) Cochlear Nuclear Synapses

167

b. Vestibular Mechanism
Describe these structures of the vestibular mechanism.
What is the general function of this mechanism?

(1) Utricle

(2) Saccule

(3) Central Structure of Labyrinth

(4) Semicircular Canals

    (a) Vertical Canals

        i) Anterior

        ii) Posterior

    (b) Horizontal Canal

c.   Inner Ear Functions

(1)   Functions for Hearing Mechanism

(a)   Basilar Membrane

i)   Frequency Analysis

ii)   Transduction
How does the basilar membrane act as an energy transducer?

(b)   Auditory Nerve

i)   Threshold
Define threshold *as it applies to auditory testing.*

ii)   Firing Rate of the Nerve
How does firing rate of the acoustic nerve relate to the listener's perception of loudness?

iii)   Frequency Perception
What is the current theory regarding the role of the auditory nerve in frequency perception?

iv)   Temporal Perception
What is meant by "temporal perception?"

(2)   Functions of Vestibular Mechanism
       Describe the significance of these aspects of
       vestibular function.
       (a)   Perception of Position in Space

       (b)   Relationship to Extraocular Muscles

       (c)   Relationship to Muscles of Posture and
              Locomotion

III.   The Central Auditory System
         In the spaces provided, describe these anatomical aspects of the central auditory system.

         A.   Location and Limits

         B.   Structures of the Central Auditory System

                1.   Brainstem Structures

                       a.   Pons

                       b.   Midbrain

                2.   Thalamus
                       What other special senses have relay centers in the thalamus?

                3.   Cerebral Cortex

                       a.   Heschl's's Gyrus

                       b.   Association Areas

C.	Functions of the Central Auditory System: The Central Auditory Pathways

Describe the course of auditory stimuli from the cochlea to the cerebral cortex via the structures listed below. How are these action potentials tracked? How do audiologists employ such tracking for diagnostic purposes? Describe any role physiologists feel it may have in refining the listener's perception of auditory stimuli.

1.	Brainstem

a.	Pons

(1)	Cochlear Nuclei

(a)	Dorsal Cochlear Nucleus

(b)	Ventral Cochlear Nucleus

i)	Anteroventral Cochlear Nucleus

ii)	Posteroventral Cochlear Nucleus

(c)	Tonotopic Representation
What is tonotopic representation?

(2)	Superior Olivary Complex

(a)	Decussation

(b)	Localization of Sound Source

b. Midbrain

  (1) Lateral Lemniscus

    (a) Inferior Colliculus

    (b) Nucleus of the Lateral Lemniscus

    (c) Olivocochlear Bundle Fibers
         *How do audiologists use action potentials
         from the olivocochlear fibers to evaluate
         cochlear functions?*

  (2) Association With Other Functions

2. Thalamus

  a. Location

  b. General Function

    (1) Sensory

    (2) Emotional

  c. Medial Geniculate Body

3. Cerebral Cortex
Does the cerebral cortex appear to deal differently with meaningful auditory stimuli than it does with non-meaningful ones?

a. Temporal Lobe

(1) Heschl's Gyrus

(2) Association Areas

(3) Interaction with Other Cortical Functions
Describe the way auditory signals are associated with signals from other input modalities at the level of the cerebral cortex.

b.   Interhemispheric Differences

    (1)   Sensation

    (2)   Perception
    Describe what is meant by "perception." Are there different levels of perception?

        (a)   Interhemispheric Differences in Auditory Perception

            i)   Perception of Speech

            ii)   Perception of Other Stimuli

    (3)   Auditory Discrimination

        (a)   Of General Acoustic Stimuli

        (b)   Of Speech Stimuli

    (4)   Auditory Memory

UNIT 7: THE AUDITORY SYSTEM
Self Test

1. The external auditory meatus is part of the _____
   _____.

2. What is the major contribution of the pinna to hearing?_____
   _____.

3. The skeleton of the distal portion of the external auditory meatus is
   composed of _____.

4. The main function of the middle ear is _____
   _____.

5. The ossicular chain is comprised of which three bones?_____
   _____.

6. Pressure equalization for the middle ear is provided by _____
   _____.

7. The semicircular canals are parts of the _____.

8. The end organ for hearing is the _____.

9. With what fluid are scala vestibuli and scala tympani filled ? _____.

10. The cranial nerve which carries sound activated nerve impulses to the
    brainstem is _____.

11. The cranial nerves connect to the central nervous system at what
    structure? _____.

12. Nerve fibers of the auditory pathways cross from one side of the brainstem
    to the contralateral side at the level of the _____
    _____.

13. In most people, meaningful language input is mediated primarily in the
    _____.

14. The auditory cortex is located in the _____.

15. The first synapses of the central auditory pathway are the _____
_____.

16. A tumor which affects transmission of VIIIth nerve impulses is called :_____
_____.

17. Indicate in which division (central or peripheral) of the auditory system the following structures are located.

a. stapedius muscle _____   f. stapes   _____

b. cochlea   _____   g. ceruminous glands   _____

c. pinna   _____   h. VIIIth nerve   _____

d. dorsal cochlear nucleus _____   i. Heschl's gyrus   _____

e. inferior olive   _____   j. organ of corti   _____

18. The semicircular canals are parts of what system? _____.

19. Which ossicle is located closest to the tympanic membrane? _____.

20. What are the three main parts of the peripheral hearing mechanism?

_____.

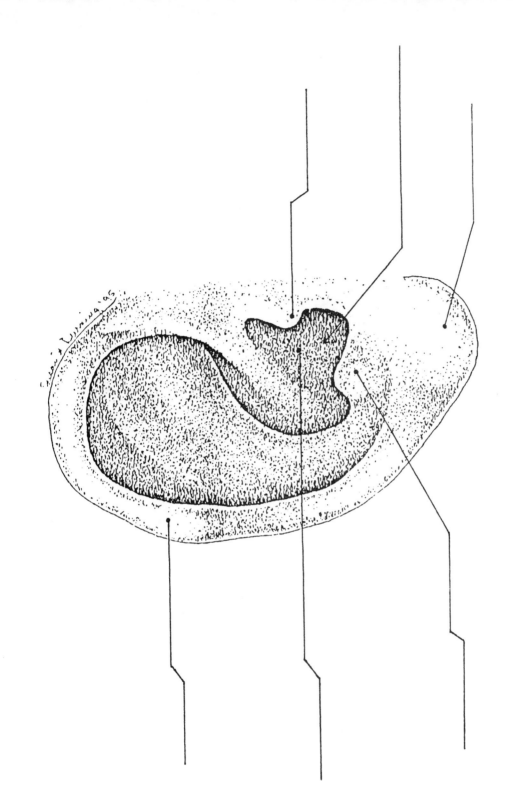

PINNA

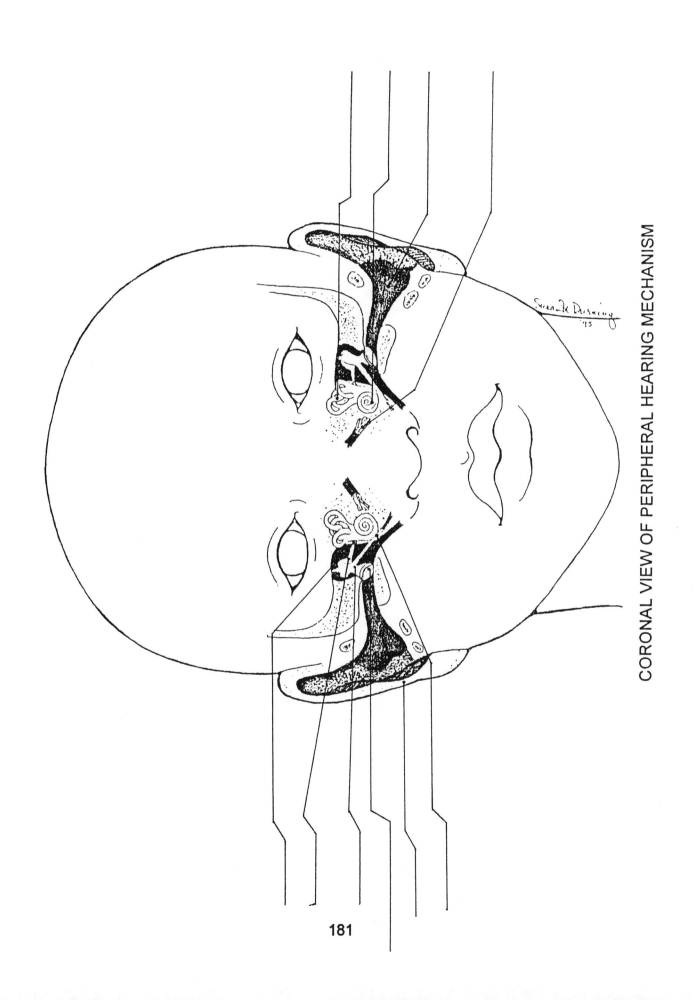

CORONAL VIEW OF PERIPHERAL HEARING MECHANISM

ANSWERS TO SELF TESTS

UNIT 1: INTRODUCTION TO ANATOMY -- ANSWERS TO SELF TEST

1.   Erect, facing the observer; front; directed toward the observer; at the sides.

2.   Physiology

3.   Coronal

4.   Transverse

5.   Superior

6.   Inferior or distal

7.   Distal

8.   Lateral

9.   Inferior or distal

10.   Anatomy

11.   Geriatric

12.   Developmental

13.   Pathologic

14.   Experimental

UNIT 2:   CYTOLOGY AND HISTOLOGY - ANSWERS TO SELF TEST

1.   Protoplasm.

2.   Growth; reproduction; metabolism; adaptation

3.   Histology.

4.   Nucleus.

5.   a)Nervous; b)Epithelial; c)Muscle; d)Connective; e)Nervous

6.   a)Ectoderm; b)Mesoderm; c)Ectoderm; d)Mesoderm;
      e)Endoderm (Entoderm).

7.   Mandible and hyoid bones; thyroid and cricoid cartilages

8.   Intake of food water and air.

9.   Germ layers

10.   Diarthrodial or synovial

11.   Striated or skeletal

12.   A motor neuron and the muscle fibers it supplies.

13.   Insertion

14.   A collection of tissues that work together to perform a specific function.

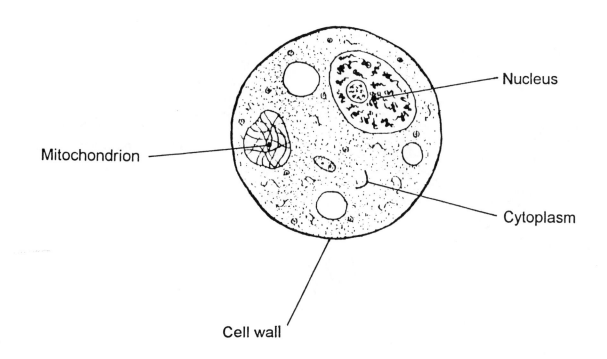

Nucleus

Mitochondrion

Cytoplasm

Cell wall

SOMATIC CELL

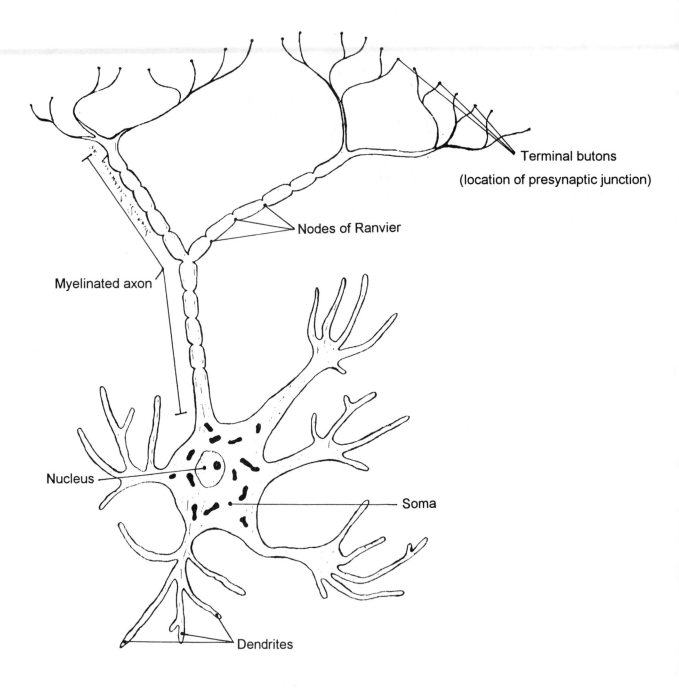

Terminal butons

(location of presynaptic junction)

Nodes of Ranvier

Myelinated axon

Nucleus

Soma

Dendrites

NEURON

UNIT 3: RESPIRATORY SYSTEM - ANSWERS TO SELF TEST

1. Chemical and Biological

2. Volume; Boyle's Law.

3. a. Upper; b. Lower; c. Upper; d. Upper; e. Upper; f. Lower; g. Lower; h. Upper; i. Lower; j. upper

4. To provide compressed air for speech

5. The lungs and the respiratory passages

6. One inhalation and one exhalation

7. 12 to 20 cycles/min.

8. The muscles of respiration

9. The diaphragm and the external intercostals

10. Relax

11. Cervical

12. Bucket handle movement

13. Forced exhalation, such as blowing

14. Sternum

15. Spirometer

16. Thoracic

17. Tidal volume

18. Vital capacity

19. .16

20. Supplemental air; can be forcefully exhaled from resting expiratory level.

21. Diaphragmatic/abdominal; thoracic.

22. Rapid, shallow cycles (tachypnea) gradually becoming longer and deeper (hyperpnea), followed by transient cessation of breathing (apnea). After this, the pattern repeats.

23. Chronic obstructive pulmonary disease (C.O.P.D.) is an irreversible condition in which the patient is unable to make optimal use of the oxygen in the air for respiration. Depending on the severity of the condition, the patient may be forced to speak in short utterances. Expiratory volume velocity may be insufficient to produce a normal voice. Since the condition is irreversible, rehabilitation goals should be aimed at accommodation instead of recovery.

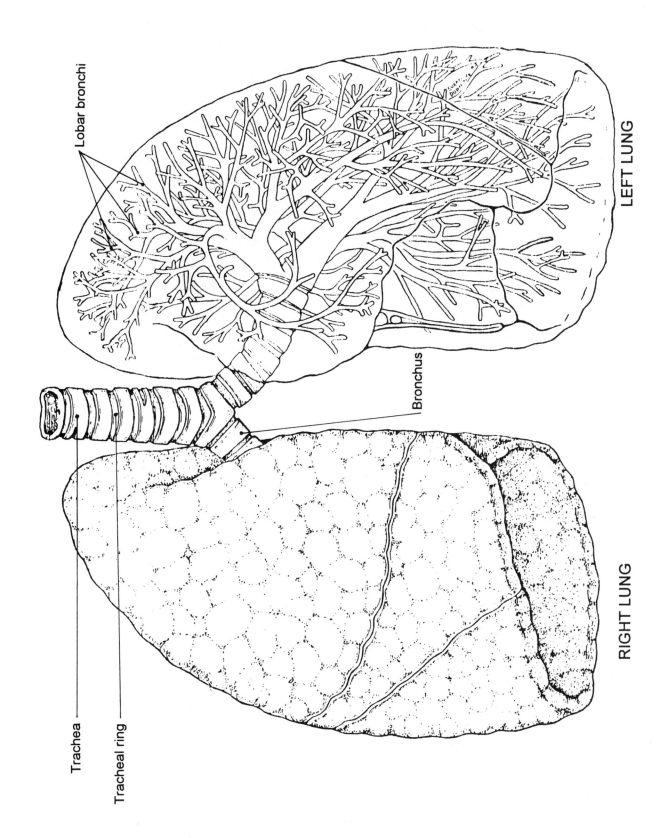

Trachea

Tracheal ring

Lobar bronchi

Bronchus

LEFT LUNG

RIGHT LUNG

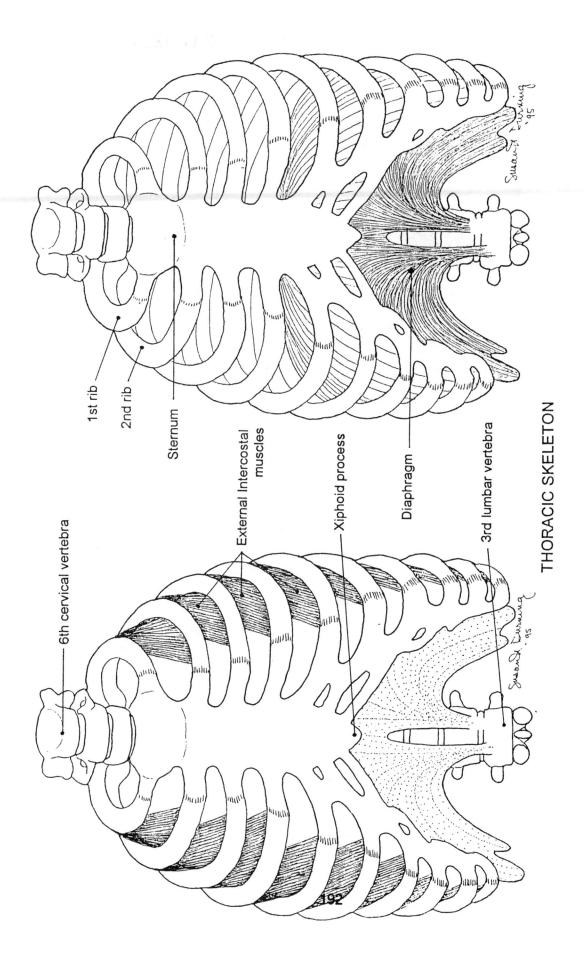

6th cervical vertebra

External Intercostal muscles

Xiphoid process

Diaphragm

3rd lumbar vertebra

1st rib

2nd rib

Sternum

THORACIC SKELETON

UNIT 4: THE PHONATORY SYSTEM - ANSWERS TO SELF TEST

1. To protect the airway.

2. Anterior

3. To produce a phonatory source for speech.

4. The complex tone produced when loosely approximated vocal folds emit pulses of pulmonary air.

5. The number of times the glottis opens and closes in a given time.

6. The amount of subglottic pressure

7. The space between the vocal folds

8. Skull

9. The thyroid cartilage

10. The cricoid cartilage

11. Laminae (sing.: lamina)

12. "Adam's apple"

13. Cricoid cartilage

14. The vocal processes of the arytenoid cartilages

15. Abduction

16. (d) Cricothyroid, thyroarytenoid and vocalis muscles

17. (a) Posterior cricoarytenoid muscles

18. The muscular processes of the arytenoid cartilages

19. Abducted

20. Synovial

21. Vocal ligament

22. The intrinsic muscles are attached to laryngeal structures at both ends, while the extrinsic muscles are attached to laryngeal structures at one end and attached to other structures (i.e., the sternum) at the other end.

23. The posterior cricoarytenoids

24. To adjust the support, posture and position of the larynx

25. Subglottic pressure

26. Approximately 210 Hz. (Some authorities give 260Hz.)

27. During phonation the glottis closes through combined myoelastic and aerodynamic forces. Myoelasticity is the tendency of the muscles to resist deformation. Aerodynamic forces result from the Bernoulli effect, or the tendency of the internal pressure of a liquid (such as air) to decrease as its velocity increases.

28. The thyroarytenoid and vocalis muscles

29. Superiorly

30. Radiologists and speech-language pathologists observe cineradiographic studies of the upper airway during deglutition to note if any of the medium collects in the valleculae.

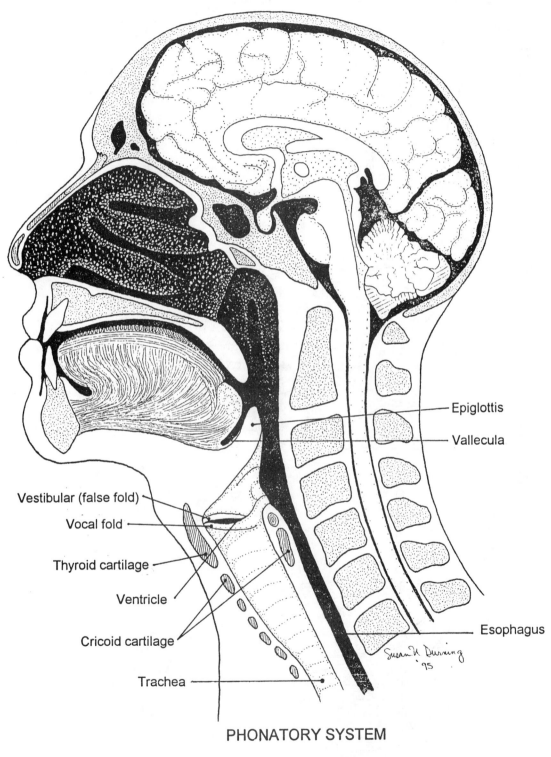

Epiglottis

Vallecula

Vestibular (false fold)

Vocal fold

Thyroid cartilage

Ventricle

Cricoid cartilage

Trachea

Esophagus

PHONATORY SYSTEM

195

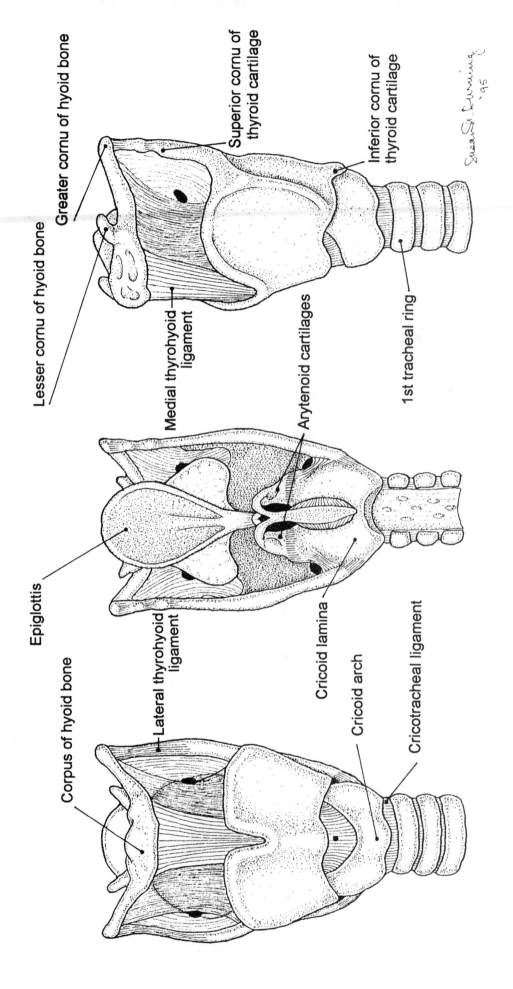

Greater cornu of hyoid bone

Superior cornu of thyroid cartilage

Inferior cornu of thyroid cartilage

Lesser cornu of hyoid bone

Medial thyrohyoid ligament

Arytenoid cartilages

1st tracheal ring

Epiglottis

Corpus of hyoid bone

Lateral thyrohyoid ligament

Cricoid lamina

Cricoid arch

Cricotracheal ligament

SKELETON OF THE LARYNX

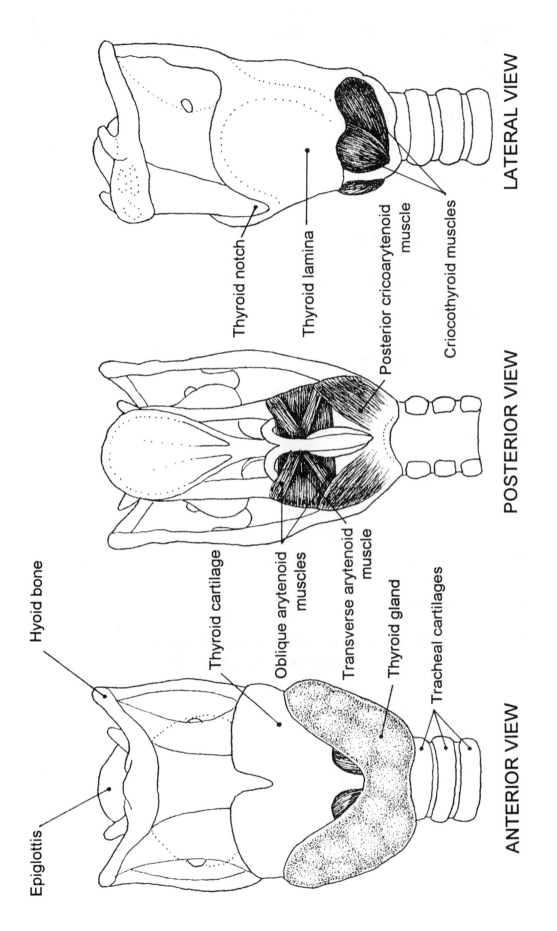

LARYNX

ANTERIOR VIEW

POSTERIOR VIEW

LATERAL VIEW

Epiglottis

Hyoid bone

Thyroid cartilage

Oblique arytenoid muscles

Transverse arytenoid muscle

Thyroid gland

Tracheal cartilages

Thyroid notch

Thyroid lamina

Posterior cricoarytenoid muscle

Criocothyroid muscles

UNIT 5: THE ARTICULATORY MECHANISM - ANSWERS TO SELF TEST

1. Cranium

2. Frontal; temporal; sphenoid; parietal; occipital

3. Zygomatic

4. Mandible

5. Oral; nasal; pharyngeal

6. (Two) orbits, the nasal cavity, and the cranial cavity

7. The forehead (frons)

8. Palatoglossus muscles

9. Tongue; velum

10. "Cleft palate"

11. Orbicularis oris

12. Oral stage

13. Temporalis; masseter; and medial (internal) pterygoid muscles

14. Velum; tongue; mandible

15. Normally, with changes in dentition, the angle decreases as the individual reaches adulthood, then increases again as age advances and dentition is lost.

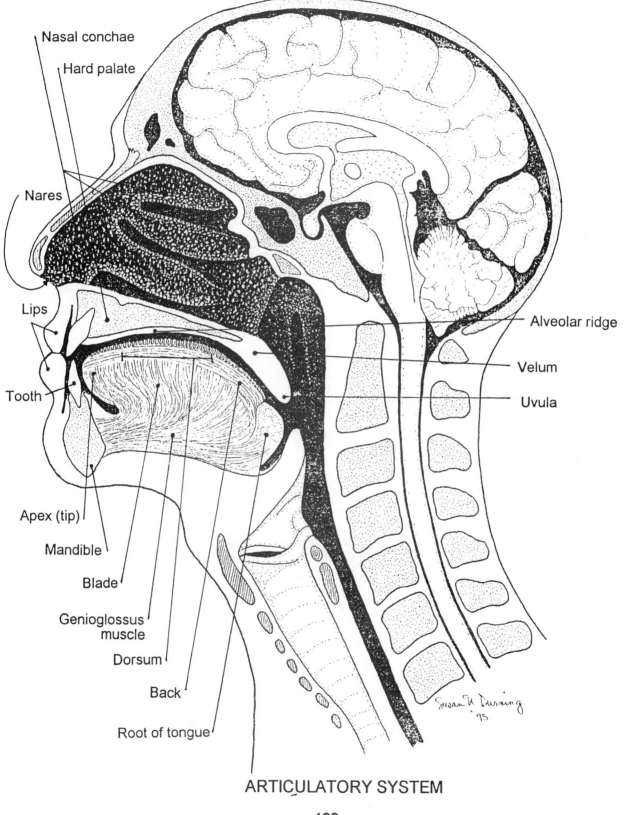

Nasal conchae

Hard palate

Nares

Lips

Tooth

Apex (tip)

Mandible

Blade

Genioglossus
muscle

Dorsum

Back

Root of tongue

Alveolar ridge

Velum

Uvula

ARTICULATORY SYSTEM

199

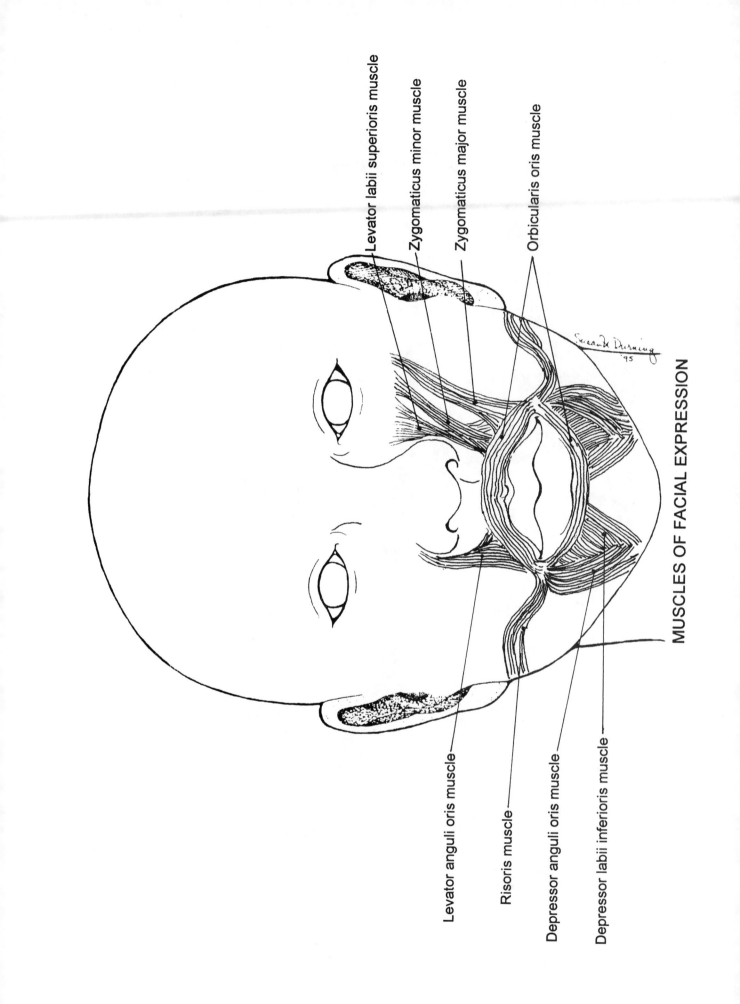

Levator labii superioris muscle

Zygomaticus minor muscle

Zygomaticus major muscle

Orbicularis oris muscle

Levator anguli oris muscle

Risoris muscle

Depressor anguli oris muscle

Depressor labii inferioris muscle

MUSCLES OF FACIAL EXPRESSION

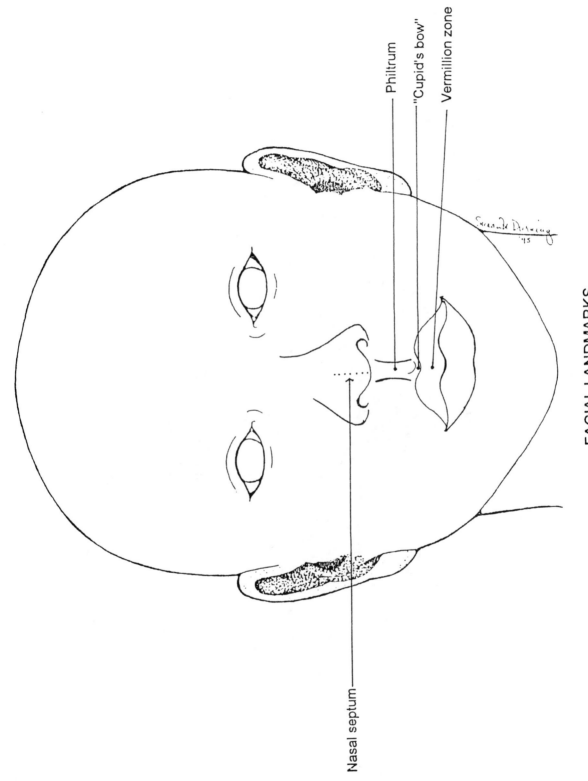

Philtrum

"Cupid's bow"

Vermillion zone

Nasal septum

FACIAL LANDMARKS

201

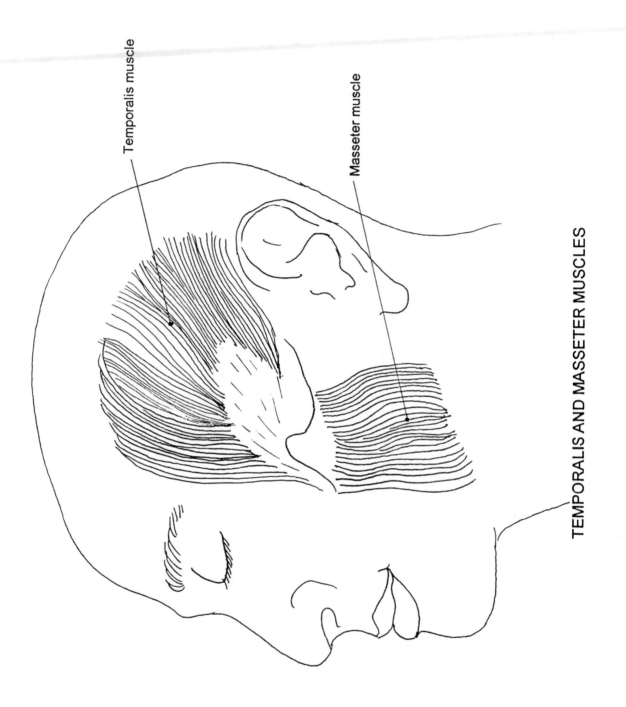

Temporalis muscle

Masseter muscle

TEMPORALIS AND MASSETER MUSCLES

202

UNIT 6: THE NERVOUS SYSTEM - SELF TEST ANSWERS

1. Central nervous system & peripheral nervous system

2. The brain and the spinal cord

3. Afferent

4. Efferent

5. Frontal

6. 12

7. Peripheral

8. Spinal & cranial nerves and autonomic nervous system

9. Sympathetic nervous system

10. The association areas of the cerebral cortex

11. Synapses

12. Gyri

13. Lateral sulcus (fissure of Sylvius)

14. Central fissure (fissure of Rolando)

15. Sensory (tactile) reception

16. Pars triangularis of the left frontal lobe

17. Homonymous hemianopsia

18. Paralysis of the contralateral musculature

19. Brainstem

20. Hypoglossal nerve (XII).

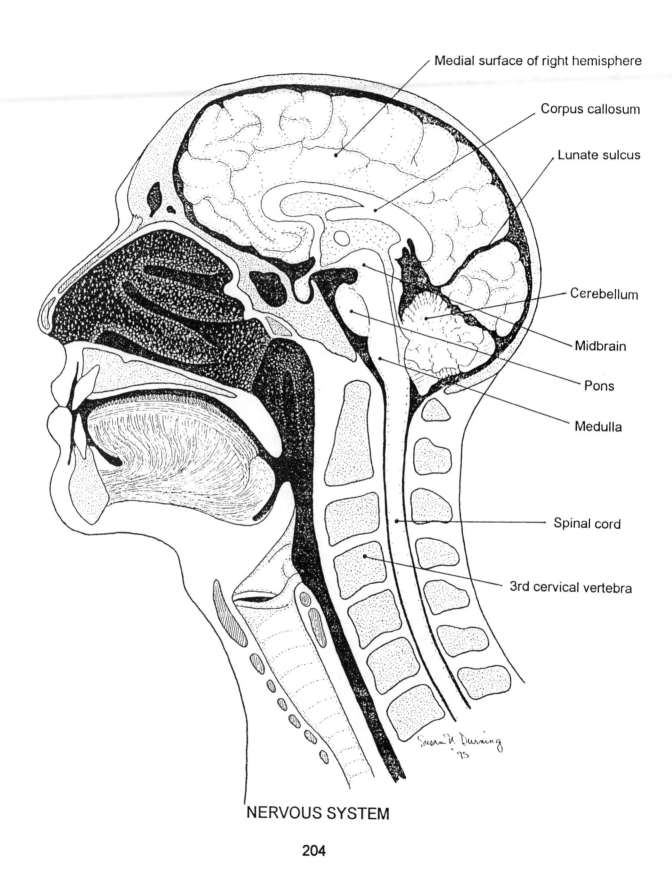

Medial surface of right hemisphere

Corpus callosum

Lunate sulcus

Cerebellum

Midbrain

Pons

Medulla

Spinal cord

3rd cervical vertebra

NERVOUS SYSTEM

UNIT 7: THE AUDITORY SYSTEM - SELF TEST ANSWERS:

1. Peripheral hearing mechanism

2. To direct acoustic energy to the external auditory meatus.

3. Cartilage

4. Match the acoustic impedance of the inner ear to that of the environment.

5. Malleus; incus; stapes

6. Eustachian (pharyngotympanic; auditory) tubes

7. Vestibular apparatus

8. Cochlea

9. Perilymph

10. Vestibulocochlear (acoustic) nerve or cranial nerve VIII

11. The pons

12. Superior olivary complex

13. Cerebral cortex of the dominant cerebral hemisphere

14. Temporal lobe

15. Cochlear nuclei

16. Acoustic neuroma

17. a) peripheral; b) peripheral; c) peripheral; d) central; e) central; f) peripheral; g) peripheral; h) peripheral; i) central; j) peripheral

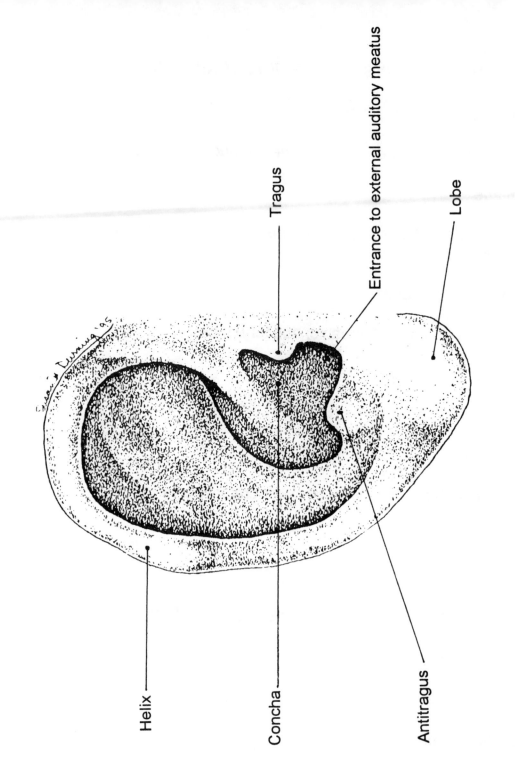

Tragus

Entrance to external auditory meatus

Lobe

Helix

Concha

Antitragus

PINNA

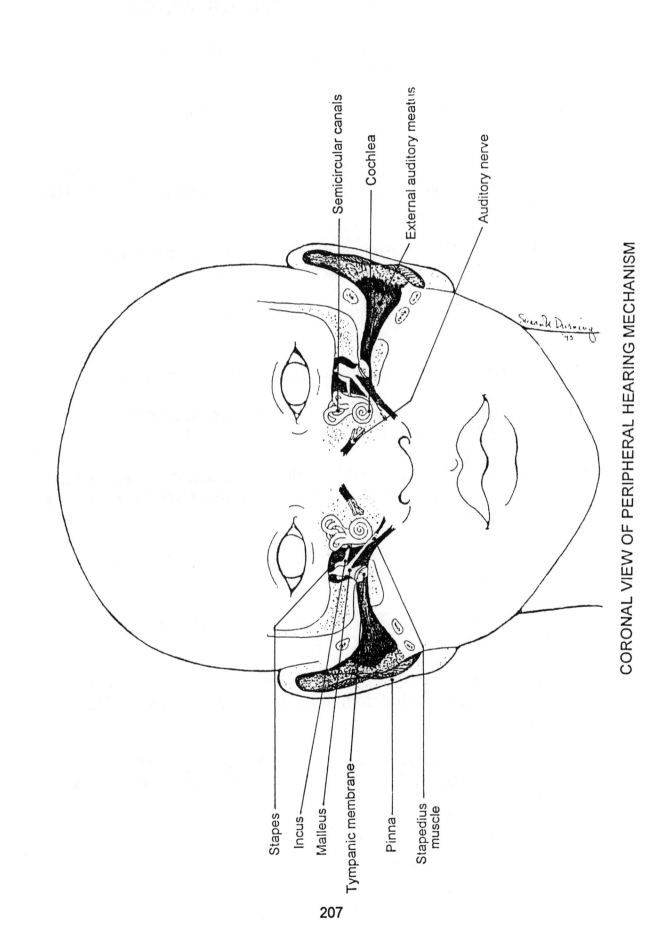

Semicircular canals

Cochlea

External auditory meatus

Auditory nerve

Stapes

Incus

Malleus

Tympanic membrane

Pinna

Stapedius muscle

CORONAL VIEW OF PERIPHERAL HEARING MECHANISM

REFERENCES and RECOMMENDED READINGS

Anderson, K. (Ed.) (1994). *Mosby's Medical, Nursing, and Allied Health Dictionary*. St.Louis: Mosby-Year Book, Inc.

Clemente, C. (1975). *Anatomy: A Regional Atlas of the Human Body*. Philadelphia: Lea & Febiger.

Daniloff, R., Schuckers, G. & Feth, L. (1980). *The Physiology of Speech and Hearing*. Englewood, Cliffs, N.J.: Prentice-Hall (Needham Heights, Ma.: Allyn & Bacon).

Hafen, B. & Karren, K. (1989). *Prehospital Emergency Care and Crisis Intervention*. Englewood, Co.: Morton Publishing.

Hamilton, W. (1977). *Textbook of Human Anatomy*. Saint Louis, Mo.: C.V. Mosby.

Katz, J. (1994). *Handbook of Clinical Audiology*. Baltimore: Willims and Wilkins.

Martin, F. (1994). *Introduction to Audiology (5th Ed.)* Englewood Cliffs, N.J.: Prentice-Hall (Needhan Heights, Ma.: Allyn & Bacon).

Minifie, F., Hixon, T. & Williams, F. (1973). *Normal Aspects of Speech, Hearing, and Language*. Englewood Cliffs, N.J.: Prentice-Hall (Needham Heights, Ma.: Allyn & Bacon).

Romanes, G. (Ed.) (1972). *Cunningham's Textbook of Anatomy, 11th ed.* London: Oxford University Press.

Thomas, C., (Ed.) (1973). *Taber's Cyclopedic Medical Dictionary*. Philadelphia: F.A. Davis Company.

Van Riper, C. & Erickson, R. (1996). *Speech Correction: An Introduction to Speech Pathology and Audiology (9th Ed.)*. Needham Heights, Ma.: Allyn & Bacon.

Zemlin, W., (1988). *Speech and Hearing Science: Anatomy and Physiology (3rd Ed.)*. Englewood Cliffs, N.J.: Prentice-Hall (Needham Heights, Ma.: Allyn & Bacon).

NOTES

NOTES

NOTES

NOTES